STRESS IN CORPORATE SECTORS AND CLINICS
INDIAN SCENARIO

PSYCHOPATHOLOGY AND AMELIORATION THROUGH COUNSELLING

STRESS IN CORPORATE SECTORS AND CLINICS
INDIAN SCENARIO

PSYCHOPATHOLOGY AND AMELIORATION THROUGH COUNSELLING

Prabal Kumar Chattopadhyay

DMSP, PhD (Clinical Psychology), NIMHANS, Bangalore University,
PhD (Clinical Psychology), Institute of Psychiatry, Maudsley Hospital,
University of London, Diplomate, I.A.B.M.C.P. (USA), Professor and
Former HOD of Psychology, Calcutta University

New Central Book Agency (P) Ltd

LONDON

HYDERABAD ERNAKULAM BHUBANESWAR

NEW DELHI KOLKATA PUNE GUWAHATI

NCBA

REGD OFFICE

8/1 Chintamoni Das Lane, Kolkata 700 009, India
email: ncbapvtltd@eth.net

OVERSEAS

NCBA (UK) Ltd. 149 Park Avenue North, Northampton, NN3 2HY, UK
email: ncbauk@yahoo.com

EXPORT

NCBA Exports Pvt. Ltd, 212 Shahpur Jat, New Delhi 110 049
email: ncbaexports@ncbapvtltd.com

BRANCHES

212 Shahpur Jat
New Delhi 110 049
email: ncbadel@ncbapvtltd.com

House No. 3-1-315, 1st Floor
Nimboliadda, Kachiguda, **Hyderabad** 500 027
email: ncbahydb@ncbapvtltd.com

Shop Nos. 3 & 4, Vinayak Towers
681/B Budhwar Peth, Appa Balwant Chowk
Pune 411 002
email: ncbapune@ncbapvtltd.com

GSS Shopping Complex, 1st Floor
Opposite College Post Office, Convent Road
Ernakulam 682 035
email: ncbaernk@ncbapvtltd.com

Shop No. 15, Bharati Towers, Ground Floor
Forest Park, **Bhubaneswar** 751 001
email: ncbabub@ncbapvtltd.com

Radhamayee Complex (Second Floor)
Opp. SBI, Panbazar, Jaswanta Road
Guwahati 781 001
email: ncbaguwahati@ncbapvtltd.com

Stress in Corporate Sectors and Clinics: Indian Scenario • Prabal Kumar Chattopadhyay

First Published: January 2014

PUBLISHER AND TYPESETTER
New Central Book Agency (P) Ltd
8/1 Chintamoni Das Lane, Kolkata 700 009

PRINTER
New Central Book Agency (P) Ltd
Web-Offset Division, Dhulagarh, Sankrail, Howrah

COVER DESIGNER
Soumen Paul

COVER PRINTER
Techno Process, Kolkata

PROOF CHECKING
Subas Maitra and Author

PROJECT TEAM
Pradip Das, Pradip Biswas, Prodip Baidya and Prabhat Jas

ISBN 978 81 7381 887 5

Price: ₹ 350.00

Dedicated to

my

Beloved Parents

Late Bankim Ch. Chattopadhyay

Late Maya Chattopadhyay

and

My Mentor

Late H. N. Murthy

and

Patients/Clients

CONTENTS

PREFACE

The present era may best be described as an era of stress. Every individual is constantly exposed to stress—no matter whether at a very personal level, or family interactional level, or occupational level, or, broadly, from a socio-cultural perspective.

Techniques applied for amelioration of stress and stress-related disorders must not aim just symptomatic relief. Treatment techniques must be oriented to symptom psychopathology. There is wide cross-cultural variations in understanding symptom psychopathology. Accordingly, intervention strategies require framing of its methodology considering cultural ingredients which prevail in symptom formation. As such, we need our own indigenous techniques for stress amelioration. Though attempts have been made during several years in India to standardise our own tests for assessment, and techniques for symptom amelioration, availability of consolidated techniques for treatment of stress-related disorders appears too meagre in comparison to the demands noted in different sectors of our life, namely, amelioration of techno-stress and those emotionally disturbed individuals who attend clinics.

The basic objective of this book is to provide a clear and concise account of the concept—stress, its related psychosocial issues, deleterious effects of stress on human health and application of remedial measures, particularly through counselling and related other behavioural measures which are indigenous in nature.

This volume has emerged from the author's frustrating experience which mounted over three decades while teaching clinical psychology at the PG level in India, on his return from abroad. Frustration occurred because—(i) the students were found to be more concerned about diagnostic labeling of the patients rather that understanding symptom psychopathology of each of the symptoms of a syndrome in context to our cultural ingredients. The latter is essential because wide cross-cultural variations exist between the Oriental and Occidental cultures and their impact on symptom manifestations in psychiatric patients; (ii) the students had to be re-oriented to find link between the symptoms of a given patient and how to consider each symptom not as a discrete phenomenon but as a whole; (iii) to motivate students to use more of indigenous psychological techniques to ameliorate the problems of our patients rather than blind borrowing of concepts—theoretical constructs which have been developed in a culturally diverse nation. Because, application of tests and techniques for amelioration developed in a culturally diverse nation is not only incomplete and ineffective but misleading too.

Of course, there had been some positive sources of inspiration to take this responsibility. These are—(i) novelty in symptom psychopathology, noted in our patients in comparison to those noted in the patients of the West, though patients of all nations—East or West—manifest same symptoms; (ii) innumerable critical issues and interesting questions raised by my students and research-scholars while applying psychotherapy or counselling on their patients/clients; (iii) over four decades of the author's clinical research experience on etiology and psychopathology of different groups of psychiatric patients have provided impetus to consolidate those data in a single write-up. The latter has enabled to cite so many case vignettes and illustrations to make the presentation readable and interesting.

With increasing need for understanding the psychosocial issues that arise in response to stress and stress-related disorders, there has been an increasing need for campaign of health promotion for the people of different age-groups. How people can cope with being at risk owing to chronic stress, and need for their awareness of the available and adequate resources have been highlighted in this treatise which definitely is a significant contribution for formulation of health promotion programme of the sufferers. Expansion of the coverage of health promotion issues and integration of the same—particularly through counselling, progressive muscular relaxation, biofeedback, and related other techniques—have been detailed in the later chapters. Also, complex relations among health hazards which arise out of stress and their management procedures have been highlighted.

In this book I have made conscious efforts to make the presentation material more interesting and relevant to cater to the need of the students and professionals. Most of the chapters depict case histories of different psychiatric patients and other highly-stressed individuals which reflect more particularly the experiences of our young generation. The presentation materials have been more directly tied to the needs of the adolescents and young adults to overcome distress which is usually found to be associated with their academic pursuit, vocational career, and material sphere of life. To avoid stress in life and to be in 'de-stress', people—both young and old—may follow the wise dictum of Rabindranath Tagore : 'TIME IS MONEY, but LEISURE IS WEALTH.'

The success of any text depends ultimately on its ability to communicate clearly to the readers and to spark interest in the field. However, writing a textbook on counselling procedure in our cultural context is a formidable task.

29 September 2013 **P. K. Chattopadhyay**

ACKNOWLEDGEMENTS

Words of Thanks.

My sincere thanks to the previous contributors on the subject—both the Indian authors and the Western authors—who have focussed upon the implications of cross-cultural variations in counselling and psychotherapy. I have duly acknowledged their contributions following standard procedure of reference citation.

I am indebted to hundreds and thousands of patients/clients and their family members who have helped me enormously to enrich my knowledge about the application of counselling techniques in context of Indian culture.

I am also thankful to the innumerable students and research fellows of mine for their queries and inquisitiveness to know about cultural impact in symptomatology, and in psychopathology of the patients. This has inspired me to prepare this treatise which provides outlines for formulation of psychopathology, counselling steps and procedures.

I express my sincere thanks and gratitude to my talented research fellow and, of late, teaching faculty of Barasat State University, Ms Deepa Shah (Das) who has spent lots of her valuable time alone for preparing the manuscript. Her excellent, scholarly feedback and suggestions have helped me to enrich the content and in its final shape. I have dearth of words to acknowledge her untiring sincere efforts and commitments.

My sincere thanks to respected Mr. Subas Maitra for his careful editing and esteemed suggestions to bring the manuscript in its published form.

I shall fail from my duty if I don't express my gratitude to my beloved parents whose passion for learning has/had motivated me to write-up this and other books.

I appreciate very much the Director, Mr. Amitabha Sen, of the New Central Book Agency (P) Ltd, Kolkata, for his instant evaluation of the content of the manuscript and approval for its publication. Also, I appreciate very much his interest in publishing many other books on psychology—to disseminate the role of psychology in different spheres of our life, particularly to enrich the student community of different allied disciplines.

I appreciate the cooperation and prompt action which I have received from the other associates of the New Central Book Agency (P) Ltd, Kolkata, for its speedy publication.

I am thankful to Mr. Manas Bhattacharjee for his careful typing and suggestions in preparing the manuscript.

Last but not least, I am indebted to Dr. (Mrs) Barna Chatterjee (Wife), Dr. Pratik Chatterjee (Son), Poulomi (Daughter-in-law), and Ramesh (My guardian) for their cooperation, patience and mental support in every step of my life.

P. K. Chattopadhyay

Chapter 1

STRESS : THE CONCEPT

The present era may best be described as an era of stress. It appears as though every individual of the present-day world is exposed to certain stress producing situations such as the threat of war, unprecedente use of nuclear energy, rapid political and economic upheaval in general, and, at a more personal level, psychological conflicts, confusions, insecurity, uncertainty, mistrust with respect to our interpersonal relationships and values and standards that one holds essential to his/her existence. Hence, a write-up on stress and its management at this stage seems appropriate. And very essential too.

Substantial advances in stress research have been made in the last few decades. This has been possible through the earliest pioneering research contributions of stalwarts like Walter Cannon (1932), Hans Selye (1956,1976) and, later, R.S. Lazarus (1968), Folkman (1997), and others. Cannon opined that when the organism experiences a threat, a heightened state of a arousal sets-in in the body. Both the sympathetic nervous system and the endocrine system get involved to mobilise the organism to either attack the threat or to flee. Hence Cannon's concept has been designated as the 'fight or flight' response. Such a motivation on the part of the organism, either to fight or to flee, in a sense, may be considered to have an adaptive value as it rescues the body from stressful exposure. On the contrary, if the organism fails either to fight or to flee and remains exposed to stress for a prolonged period of time, the heightened state of physiological arousal is likely to continue unabated, laying the groundwork for medical problems in the organism over time. For example, prolonged secretion of hydrochloric acid (HCL) in the stomach can cause formation of ulcers.

Hans Selye (1956, 1976) developed the concept of 'General Adaptation Syndrome' (GAS) which consists of three phases, namely, alarm phase, stage of resistance, and stage of exhaustion. The GAS is basically an outcome of Selye's prolonged research on animals applying different types of stressors. Initially though Selye intended to focus on the impact of sex hormone in stress reaction, later he advocated that all stressors—regardless of type—lead to an enlargement of adrenal cortex, thus stressors produce essentially the same pattern of physiological responses. The GAS focuses upon the interplay of physiological and environmental factors in stress reaction. Whereas Cannon's work explored primarily adrenomedullary responses to stress, particularly catecholamine secretion, Selye's work more closely focussed upon adrenocortical responses to stress. Furthermore, Selye's concept postulates a physiological mechanism which underlie in stressillness relationship. Prolonged stress can cause damage to the organism which later gets manifested in symptoms. For example, immune-related deficiencies, skeleto-muscular diseases, cardiovascular diseases, and so on.

Unlike the recent models, the earlier models of stress as those of the above have by and large ignored any significant role of psychclogical factors in stress experience. Later contributors—namely R.S. Lazarus & Folkman (1984)—advocated that in any appraisal of stress, psychological meanings of the events as well as the personality of the individual who experiences the stressful events are to be considered as important determinants. As such, question arises, how responses to stress could be uniformed? Recent research evidences reveal that particular stressors produce distinct endocrinological responses (Appley and Trunbull, 1986; Mason, 1974, 1975). Moreover, we need to consider that there are wide individual variations in the experience of stress, such as, some manifests behavioural reactions at the early stage of stressful experience, whilst some others try to swallow the distress with least behavioural gestures, and still some others experience many of the debilitating effects of stress event in anticipation of occurrence of stress. Therefore, evaluation of stress behaviour has to depend largely onto the perceptions, biological contributions (Lazarus & Folkman, 1984; Moos, 1984), and personality dispositions of the individual, no matter what could be the type of stressor a given individual is exposed to. The early stress research was conducted on animals, and that could be the reason for such substantial missing of emphasis on human psychological factors in stress evaluation.

Psychological Model of Stress

Psychological stress is the response to situations in which one experiences threat out of a feeling that his resources—both potential and already existing ones—are ineffective. When an individual is confronted with an unexpected event or situation, he becomes engaged automatically with a rigorous cognitive exercise for appraisal of the event. Such appraisal is primarily determined by the meaning he attributes to the event he confronts. Accordingly, events may be perceived by him as positive, negative or neutral. Therefore, a given individual's perception of an event and the corresponding meaning he attributes to it are the determining factors of stress experience for him—whether or not that event is alarming, harmful and thus stressful to others. Such a process, an individual is engaged in, in evaluating the event is called 'primary appraisal' by Lazarus and Folkman (1984).

What is considered 'primary appraisal' in the psychological model of stress seems akin to that of the concept of Pavlov's 'investigatory' (Pavlov, 1927) or '*what-it-is reflex*' which, later, has been known as orienting reaction (Razran, 1961) in the physiological model of stress. To decide upon action to be taken to save oneself from the threat depends not only on the intensity of the harmful stimulus but also on the coping resources the individual possesses, and strength of its self-confidence required to apply adequate coping strategies. The latter process— i.e., self-evaluation of one's own resources and self-confidence—is called 'secondary appraisal' of the situation. Thus the whole process is an outcome of one's subjective experience/perception of the magnitude of the event and of one's own strength to cope with, whereby the individual maintains a balance between the 'primary appraisal' and 'secondary appraisal' of the event to determine its meaning and consequent action-orientation plan.

Needless to mention that when magnitude of the stress is high and required coping ability is low, substantial threat is felt (Tomaka, Blascovich *et al*, 1993). Therefore stress responses involve not only physiological reactions but psychological reactions too, viz., cognitive exercise, emotional grilling, and behavioural consequences. For example, Mr. X, aged 25 yrs, BE, unmarried, only son of the family, and Mr. Y, aged 24 yrs, B. Tech., unmarried, only son of the family—both were employees of a Grade I corporate organisation. Both of them came for receiving counselling services to the organisation's clinical psychologist (author) with the complaints of insomnia, easy irritability, and aggression. Though they came separately for individual counselling session (neither of them knew that the other was also receiving counselling services) and on enquiry it was revealed that they were posted in the same project with the supervision of the same boss. Both of them reported separately that they have been bullied by the boss, whom they described as angry, biased with racial feelings, and abuses the associates in presence of others and that too using unparliamentary words. Both of them were threatened by the boss that they may be victimised in their next interim assessment. Both of them were reported to be sincere and till date their interim assessment records were satisfactory. None of them reported any other sources of stress in their life, viz., home, friends, etc. The former client was very much upset with the boss's attitude and took it as an insulation (ego-threat to him) so much so that he decided to leave the job. Actually he wanted to get rid of the boss—not the job. The latter client did not decide to leave the job but was feeling uneasy and disturbed as his aggression used to get displaced frequently. On further enquiry, it was revealed that the boss had shown same type of attitude to other senior colleagues also. The latter client desired even to go for confrontation with that boss but, remaining indecisive in this respect, he came for counselling assistance. It is clear from the above example that the same event had been perceived stressful to both the clients but with different magnitude and reactions. The former desired to take avoidance coping while the latter took fighting strategy for coping. The latter said, "I've earned the job myself. I won't leave the job." However, counselling helped both of them to be with the same boss and same job with comfortable feelings.

Physiological Model of Stress

Advances in stress research has been possible through research on the psychophysiology of stress (Chattopadhyay, 1980, 1983, 1990, 1995, 2008), namely, the links between stress and corticosteroid functions, factors which influence the release of endogenous opiod peptides and their links to the human immune system, individual temperamental differences in nervous system activity, e.g., sympathetic and parasympathetic, and 'individual organ specificity' (Lader & Wing, 1966) and 'response specificity' (Lader & Wing, 1966) in stress response as could be revealed through physiological measures—EEG, GSR, heart-rate, blood pressure and so on. This has helped us understanding the pathways by which stress exerts adverse effects on health.

When we experience stress, our brain sends signals to the endocrine system along two major pathways (Dallman, Bhatnagar and Viau, 2000). The first pathway is rooted through the autonomic nervous system (ANS). The sympathetic division of the ANS gets activated through the hypothalamus which involves stimulation of the central part of the adrenal gland, called adrenal medulla, Consequently large amount of catecholamines is released into our blood stream; our body is mobilised for action (Lundberg, 2000), owing to such catecholamine elevation. For example, increased respiration rate, heart rate, high blood pressure and sweat gland activity. As a result, we become alert/vigilant to react to stimuli. Likewise dilatations of the pupils of our eyes increase our visual sensitivity (Weiten & Lloyd, 2004). The sympathetic nervous system's activation stimulates the adrenal glands, which releases epinephrine and norepinephrine. These catecholamines produce the 'keyed-up' feeling (Hecker and Thrope, 2005) we experience when we are under severe stress.

The second pathway involves more direct communication between the brain and the endocrine system. Receiving signals from the hypothalamus, the pituitary glands secrete ACTH (adrenocorticotropic hormone) and stimulate the outer part of the adrenal glands called the adrenal cortex. Such stimulation, in turn, helps releasing corticosteriods. The latter hormones increase our energy and ward-off tissue inflammation in case of injury (Munck, 2000; Hecker and Thorpe, 2005).

Impact of prolonged and severe stress is always injurious to our health—no matter whether stress originates from within or due to conflicts in social interaction, or due to family misunderstanding, or due to work-place dissatisfaction. Of course, these sources are mutually intertwined with each other. Since the present write-up is on organisational stress, the next chapter will be devoted to the source of work stress.

Chapter 2

SOURCES OF WORK STRESS

Stress occurs in a wide range of circumstances. For evaluation of work stress and its management one has to focus equally upon the factors related to both the employer and the employee. Stress results from a mismatch (Leka and Griffiths, 2003) between the expectation of the employer and the employee, i.e., due to a mismatch in the demand-supply ratio, where normally employers stand on the demand side and employees are the suppliers. Of course, in certain cases, the reverse may also be true where the employees show grievances due to their unmet expectations where the organisation fails to reciprocate as per their commitments. The sources of work stress may broadly be discussed under the following heads :

(1) **Human factors**

(a) Attitude and mode of interaction of the employers toward their employees.

(b) The employees' personality characteristics, emotional predisposition, and coping skills.

(c) Family-work organisation interface.

(2) **The work and the work environment**

1. Human factors

(a) **Employer's perspectives**

(i) **Attitude and mode of interaction of the employers toward their employees**—Of the different organisational sources of stress, attitudinal deficits are most important. Angry supervisors who do not think twice to be brutal to the employees (Nowack and Wimer, 2011) induce stress in the latter. Such supervisors are result-oriented with a desire to make employees similarly result-oriented and hence they are constantiy highly vigilant. They usually use harsh words with a fault-finding tendency in the employees. Their impression is that only through punishment they can increase total work-output of the organisation no matter whether the employees feel mentally perturbed. In some cases perceived inequalities are reported by the employees regarding bias in the supervisors' attitude towards some particular race or religion of the employees. In some instances, bullying the employees and even sexual harassments are reported (Nowack and

Wimer, 2011). Such supervisors have been designated as "toxic" and "interpersonally challenged" by Nowack and Wimer (2011). From such dealings the employees develop a sense of low confidence in self, resulting in associated symptoms like isolation and inadequacy. Physical complaints, namely sleep disturbance, high blood pressure, gastric irritation in the stomach, etc. are reported. All these fit into the diagnosis of clinical depression. Behaviourally, employees are found to be easily irritable, non-cooperative and stubborn.

(ii) **Concern of the supervisors about the work output of the organisations vis-a-vis total welfare of the employees**—Work-oriented supervisors usually remain unconcerned about the mental health of the employees. They believe in the principle of 'Hire & Fire'. They fail to understand that such change in the employees, in the long run, would hamper the constant progress of the total turnover of the organisation. Instead, to keep pace with the competitive market, it would be much profitable if experienced workers could be provided with required emotional support so that they can exert themselves with full motivation out of their attachment with the organisation as well as for their secured future prospect.

In contrast, some supervisors may be interpersonally very easy going too cosy, but remain totally unconcerned about the work progress of the employees vis-a-vis annual turnover of the organisation. Such a situation is also equally distressing to the employees. So, work stress does not necessarily mean heavy work schedule—absence of required schedule is also equally stressful. For example, in R & D sections of several organisations —where supervisors do not provide adequate supervision to and concern about the trainees' progress of work—it is found that the trainees become frustrated and depressed. Though the trainees may be receiving financial support from the respective organisation, lack of concern of the supervisors about the trainees' future prospect make them less creative and financial packages they receive no longer act as 'incentives' for them. Such indifferent attitude of the supervisors 'eats away' (Nowack and Wimer, 2011) creativity and talent of the trainees/employees, they, out of frustration, decide to 'quit' (Nowack and Wimer, 2011). On enquiry it is revealed that such a self-motivation to quit develops in the employees not because they want to leave the job, they rather want to get rid of the environment and/ or the supervisors as because the trainees' trust and confidence onto the organisation have declined significantly. This creates damage to the organisations' annual turnover on the one hand, and destroys 'citizenship behavioural' attachment (Rousseau, 2004) of the employees towards the organisations on the other.

(iii) **Whether work can retain well the employees' values and ethical standards**—It is highly stressful if the job requires employees to do certain things that go against their values and norms. Such a pressure may be created by the organisation on the employees directly or indirectly. For example, in the former to expect from an employee to assist in the boss's personal works, namely, household management, and so on, while, in the latter, instigation from the employer and thereupon to make it conditional that the employees' promotion would be subject to the employer's need satisfaction, viz., sexual encounterment and so on. Individuals with an assertive type of personality may protest, or else, out of fear of loss of job the concerned employee may be compelled to present a false self in satisfying the demand of the boss. It incurs a significant cost in the employees emotionally which can be insidious to physical and mental health later in life (Nowack and Wimer, 2011).

(iv) **Lack of support providing attitude of the organisation**—Employees have expectations to receive support from their colleagues, particularly from the supervisors, when they face hurdles in work place (Leka and Griffiths, 2003). If supervisors and colleagues can realise such a need of the employees and can provide necessary support to them, many a times intensity of stress can be reduced to a minimum (Leka and Griffiths, 2003). The more the support the employees get, the lesser the experience of stress they report.

Associates—Unpleasant, non-cooperative (Nowack and Wimer, 2011), mischievous co-workers can cause severe work stress. Contrarily, a team-spirit is expected to prevail in the work environment. Collaboration fosters positive mood and pro-social behaviour which are essential to ameliorate work-stress and to enhance productivity. Stress emanating from social environment and out of political issues in the work conditions is not only unhealthy and harmful to one's life, but undesired too.

(v) **If the organisation is not concerned about the opportunities that would be provided to the employees for their career development**—Stagnancy in work position, i.e., deprived of promotion for a long time, would create frustration in any employee. Organisations should take care of timely promotional prospect. Of course, promotional prospect depends not only upon the employer but on the employees also. From the latter's point of view one should have a sound-work evaluation record viz., satisfactory performance with regularity, punctuality, and in involvement with the work vis-a-vis with the organisation. From the former's point of view there must be unbiased performance evaluation system, and fair deals in offering promotion to a committed worker. If possible, to provide opportunities to the employees for higher education, and further training for knowledge-refreshing; also organisations be unbiased in placement for onsite projects, and so on.

(vi) **When employees are deprived of recreational facilities in the work environment**—This is very much required to overcome fatigue, monotony and to acquire more work energy and also to release tension and worries. Such facilities be provided particularly for break-times and after-hours free times. Nowadays some of the organizations, namely, corporates, do provide recreational facilities but boss's attitude sometimes create hindrance on the part of the employee to avail of that benefits. My experience in counselling with the employees of the corporate organisations show that joining gym even at break-times has created threat in the employee by the boss to the extent of submitting negative remarks in the employee's confidential report. This created further tension and less motivation for that worker where 1 or 2 such workers decided to leave the job. So, employees do not want to leave the job as such but want to get rid of the boss (Nowack & Wimer, 2011). Contrarily, in one or two cases, this has also come to my notice that with the plea of joining for recreational activities, viz., gym, within the organisational premises itself, the concerned employee has created certain adverse environmental situation in the work place, through drug abuse, teasing, and so on, for which matters the boss has to had take drastic actions.

Recreational activities—weak-end meets and several social events—be extended for the family members of the workers too. The latter can help not only to combat stress but also can buffer stress by providing opportunities to bridge the gap in relationship that occurs with the family members. Owing to the workers' shift duty schedule and in some cases due to unscheduled work pressure e.g., sudden tour programme, the workers fail to provide at least minimum required time for their family members.

(vii) **When employees are deprived owing to lack of opportunities to participate in decision-making policies of the organisation**—Every individual has a need to control, depending upon the nature of the work one is assigned to, and the position he holds in the organisation. If management pays attention to fulfil such a psychological need of the employee that provides a 'we' feeling in the employees it, in turn, reduces their tension and insecurity. For example, access to participate in policy-making issues related to job hours, nature of rotations, shift arrangement, job placement, and designing, problem-solving and matters related to work place environment and so on that enables one to exercise his cognitive potentialities and also to satisfy his leadership qualities. This enhances work motivation, work involvement (Tekleab & Taylor, 2003), and dedications to the organisation (Nowack & Wimer, 2011), and reduces grievances against the organisation. Workers who cannot participate in the decision-making show higher rates of absenteeism, job dissatisfaction and poor job performance (Leka & Griffiths, 2005). Increase in absenteeism and persistent high stress enhances release of hormones (Nowack & Wimer, 2011) which gets associated with adverse health, such as hypertension, cardiovascular diseases, and so on.

One might argue that direct participation of the employees may prompt them for 'grumbling when they will be informed of bad news' (Nowack & Wimer, 2011), e.g., loss of production and financial recession, In this context Nowack & Wimer (2011) are of the opinion the 'grumbling would be better compared to the suppressed resentment, if employees feel that they have been kept in dark'.

Also to see that group representatives from different sections of workers can have access to information related to the annual turnover of the organisation. This prepares the workers mentally ready to share the burden, if any, on part of the organisation. Knowledge of the 'end-result' acts as a reinforcement to the worker at least psychologically which is essential in building and maintaining 'psychological contract' (Rousseau, 2004) with the organisation.

The concept and necessity of maintaining psychological contract and how it gets violated due to organisation's attitude to the workers will be discussed later in this chapter.

(viii) **Feedback**—On completion of the work, be it complex or simple, the concerned worker possesses a psychological demand within, that he/she would be provided with feedback. Positive feedback acts as reinforcement while only negative feedback without any concrete suggestions for improvement of quality of work erodes self-confidence and demotivates the workers. Sometimes supervisors/bosses do not bother to receive feedback about their leadership style and its impact on the interpersonal interaction of the workers.

Feedback, on the one hand, helps workers to reevaluate their own potentialities and limitations and, on the other, it provides them a feeling that each one's contribution has an impact into the annual turnover of the organisation. The latter reduces stress and provides a feeling of bondage with the organisation. It has tremendous impact on the mental health of the employees and productivity of the organisation.

(ix) **When management is not concerned about organisational dysfunctions and uncared about its adverse impact onto the associates**—Loss of care and concern for the employee creates a 'burnout' experience (Leiter & Maslach, 2001) in them. Job burnout is a syndrome which constitutes of feelings of reduced personal accomplishment, poor interpersonal contact, emotional exhaustion and even depersonalisation in some cases. Unpleasant, non-cooperative workers drag down both the well-being and productivity of the organisation (Nowack & Wimer, 2011).

Job burnout in recent years is reaching extreme levels due to the effects of organisational downsizing, job restructuring and greater concern of the organisations with the total turnout rather than employee of morale and loyalty (Gerrig & Zimbardo, 2005). Burnout leads to greater absenteeism and low turnover, impaired job performance, poor interpersonal relationship with co-workers, personal health problems, and family problems also (Maslach *et al.* 2001). Employees perceive this as violation of 'psychological contract' (Rousseau, 2004; Nowack & Wimer, 2011; Robinson & Morrison, 2000) which they had in their mind at least implicitly at the time of getting associated with the given organisation.

Psychological Contract

The concept of psychological contract (PC) was first introduced by Chris Argyris (1960) and Hary Levinson (1962). PC is an implicit contract between an individual and his organisation. The contract specifies what each expects to give and receive from the other in their relationship. PC is distinct from expectations. The latter refers simply to what the employee expects to receive from his/her employer. The PC, on the other hand, reside—like beauty in the 'eyes of the beholder' (Robinson & Rousseau, 1994) which entails a belief in what the employer is obliged to provide, based on perceived promises of reciprocal exchange (Conway & Briner, 2005). PC breach has a negative effect on performance of employees (Restubog *et al*, 2006). Unlike the formal employment contracts, PC is not made once, rather it is revised throughout the employees tenure in the organisation. The longer the relationship endures, the broader is the array of contributions and inducements that might be included in the contract (Robinson & Rousseau, 1994). PC is based on 'trust' which attempts to develop "people building" rather than "people using" organisation (Schalk & Rousseau, 2001). In the Indian scenario, Bhatnagar (2007) advocated that PC has an organisational purpose. It connotes involvement, commitment, enthusiasm and focussed effort and energy. It has both attitudinal and behavioural components.

Violation of PC

PC violation occurs when one party in such a relationship perceives another to have failed to fulfil promised obligations (Tekleab & Taylor, 2003). Since PC is based on 'trust' and involve reliance of two parties on each other, violation of PC can lead to serious psychological consequences and associated behavioural problems for the parties involved (Tekleab & Taylor, 2003). Both affective and cognitive components get involved in PC violation. For example, feeling of turnover or quitting is an effective response (Lester *et al*, 2002; Lepine *et al*, 2002) which is generally associated with PC violation (Ang. *et al*, 2003). Cognitive component includes employees' perception of employer's inducement towards them. Perception is influenced by the individual's personality trait (Raja *et al*, 2004; Rousseau, 2004; Nikolaou *et al*, 2007). If, however, certain types of people are predisposed to the perception of violation, it would be useful for managers to identify their problem so that it is addressed properly (Delcampo, 2007).

In India perspective Dhar (2009) reported that cynicism develops in the employee due to PC violation.

In sum : Attitude of the organisation including staff and their interaction with each other reflect what type of culture prevails (Leka & Griffiths, 2005) in a given organisation. Culture here means whether staff and management have developed sharing attitude in respect to their organisation's well and woes and also about their benefits and value systems. This creates a climate of openness and honesty. Frank expressions and collaborations reduce each other's tendency to retaliate (Nowack & Wimer, 2011).

(b) **Employees' perspectives**

(i) **The employees' personality characteristics, emotional predisposition, and coping skills**—Personality characteristics, in context of perception of stress, refer to those which could be considered as cardinal features of one's life. These features are persistent and consistent across time and situation. These characteristics act as stress buffers in all domains of life and not restricted to any selected sphere.

Long before, behavioural scientists, in their efforts to identify psychological risk factors for cardiovascular diseases, identified a behavioural style termed the 'Type A' behaviour pattern. Consequently, Type A behaviour pattern was formulated by two physicians,—Friedman and Rosenman (1974). As behavioural and emotional markers of such personality they identified aggressiveness, uneasing, achievement striving, time urgency, strong sense of responsibility, higher level of job involvement, hospitality, and inability to relax. The relaxation provides a sense of guilt in them as if relaxation means waste of time. They may also jeopardise their home lives by failing to spend sufficient time with their family members and their relationship with others may be more strained and difficult as they are very selective about colleagues and friends. This is because they find it difficult to cope in situations that require slow and broad focus of attention for long time (Matthews, 1982). Type A individuals fit the stereotype of coronary-prone individual. They may suppress symptoms which they experience during work and thus be unaware of the cues their body provides them to slow down. Thus they have potential risk factors for cardiovascular diseases. 'Type B' refers to those who do not possess this type of personality.

Later researchers have criticised this concept of Type A, because not all Type A individual are victims of cardiovascular diseases, though they may be related to poor health generally (Adler & Matthews, 1994). Specifically, hostility is strongly implicated as a risk factor of coronary heart disease (CHD) than are the other dimensions of Type A behaviour (Smith, 1992). There too, a particular type of hostility, viz., cynical hostility, characterised by resentment, antagonism, distrust with others and frequent anger is evident. As a result they fail to make effective use of social support from their environment (Lepore, 1995). There is an adaptive side to Type A behaviour too. This is because they can have higher occupational mobility as excellent achievers in life. Accordingly, recently, Type A behaviour has been subdivided into two categories, viz., good or 'hardy' Type A, and bad "less hardy' Type A. Highly stressed but healthy executives have multifaceted personality style, which Kobasa (1979) termed 'hardiness'. Some of the executives high in hardiness and also high in stress, Kobasa found, reported relatively few illnesses than those who reported more illnesses. Later many researchers supported Kobasa who also found that hardiness relates to both good physical and mental health (e.g., Florian, Mikulincer & Taubman, 1995).

Whether there exists any gender differences with respect to Type A behaviour and related physical and psychological illness? Realtively less number of studies on women executives have been reported in the literature so far. MacDougall, Dembroski & Krantz (1981) reported that in response to standard laboratory stressors (e.g., immersion in cold water), the cardiovascular reaction of Type A women was the same as that for Type B women. When the stressors were changed to interpersonal stressor of a competitive nature, differences were noted between the two female groups. On oral history quiz, Type A women showed greater heart rate and higher systolic blood pressure than those of Type B women. Otherwise, like that of Type A men, Type B women (nurses) showed a greater association between serum cholesterol and time-pressure, role conflict, work over load and systolic blood pressure. Based on available literature, and my personal experience for last decades with corporate organisations, it may be concluded that Type A has similar effects for men and women when they deal with stressors. However, particularly for working women, apart from their endocrinological/metabolic disturbances, viz., menstrual, and menopausal disturbances, demanding family responsibilities, working with an unsupportive boss, living with a dishonest husband and lack of job mobility and shifting duty schedule, specially overnight work, etc. increase women's risk factors for coronary disease. Overall, Type A (less with hardiness) appears to be bad for women's health as it is for those of men.

Coping Strategies—Coping refers to specific ways of perceiving, interpreting and acting when an individual is required to face stressors. Selection of coping strategies largely depends upon the personality characteristics of a given individual. Because stressor, per se, is not important in deciding upon strategy; the individual's perception of the event, and evaluation of its magnitude, the techniques he/she employs to deal with the situation are important, factors for deciding upon strategy. Aim of coping is to help minimising the experience of threat and, thereby, to reduce the heightened level of arousal caused due to confrontation with the stressors. The best coping model would be that which encourages an individual to develop certain strategies which could be considered cardinal features of his personality. Cardinal, because such techniques can be utilised by him for dealing with stress in any domain of life, not particularly work stress (e.g., managerial stress).

Cardinal features of personality include—(1) primary forces, and (2) secondary forces. The latter refers to, e.g., habit development, i.e., to be careful to regular intake of balanced diet, time management and time budgeting for physical exercise, like walking, meditation, attending gym, time schedule for restful sleep and related other matters. Also, time schedule is required for hobby, mini-vacations in between busy work schedule, and at least once a year to arrange for a tour with family members, and so on. Utilisation of secondary forces depends upon the primary forces of personality.

Primary forces mean those characteristics which designate a person as 'hard' (Kobasa, 1979). Hardiness is composed of the following characteristics—(a) Commitment, (b) Control, (c) Challenge—known as 3Cs (Kobasa & Puccetti, 1983; Nowack, 1989; Florian, Mikulinear & Taubman, 1995).

Commitment : It leads to involvement. Unless committed, one cannot get involved in any situation, be it work, family, interpersonal interaction and large social institutions. Commitment develops out of belief onto oneself, i.e., who one is, what he aims to do, and what he is doing in actuality. Family environment and childhood upbringing process have significant contributions to the development of belief in one self.

Control : It develops out of self-trust. Self-trust provides confidence which is required for both initiation and execution of task assigned to him, with full responsibility. He can influence the whole course of events, and can assume responsibility for the antecedents and consequences of the events that would occur—which doesn't depend upon luck or fate.

Challenge : Refers to a belief that change represents opportunities for growth. Persons with challenge seek new experiences, undertake change to satisfy their cognitive flexibility; they have tolerance for ambiguity. Challenge provides thrill to confront new activities with a view to learn more. They are not ready to succumb to adverse effects.

Of late, Nowack & Wimer (2011) have added a fourth 'C' to it, that is 'connection'. Workers who can easily discuss their work related issues to others (may be at times personal issues as well to close friends) and can find ways and means to keep pace with the demands on the work competition, can mitigate better the effects of stress.

In sum : Hardy individuals are likely to appraise stressful life events more favourably than those who are non-hardy. This is because the latter are predisposed to show negative effects like depression, anxiety, hostility. Thus hardiness reflects absence of negative thought and activity (Funk, 1992). They can take more direct action onto the situations which demand them to react. They are, therefore, able to apply effective active coping strategies such as, problem-focussed coping (PFC) instead of avoiding the situation which causes stress in them (Williams, Wiebe & Smith, 1992). Active coping is possible as they are mentally ready to utilise both their personal resources as well as the rescue factors (external resources) available to fight with the event/situation. As a result they can transform potentially stressful events into less stressful ones and thereby can reduce risk factors for illness. For example, executives who are high in hardiness can save themselves from risk factors of illness, viz., coronary heart disease, even when they are under severe stress because of such stress-buffering effects (Cohen & Edwards, 1989).

Use of PFC requires optimism in the individual who is under stress. Optimism is a predictor of positive coping efforts, namely symptom reduction, better adjustment to illness, and recovery from surgery including coronary artery by-pass, as it provides a positive undefeated approach to life (Scheier, Carver & Bridge, 1994). Contrarily, pessimism leads to early onset of depression even in middle-aged individuals (Bromberger & Matthews, 1996) and to cancer mortality to the elderly (Schulz, Bookwala Knapp *et al*, 1996). Individuals with optimism are high in self-esteem and low in self-denigration than those of the pessimists.

Individuals with a personality to fight rather than to fly-off of the stress-arousing situations can show a better coping, as such coping provides a long-lasting effect with less possibilities of symptom recurrence. This is because the former wants to deroute the source, whilst the latter provides a temporary relief through suppression of the event. Flying-off tendency prompts one to choose indirect resources, e.g., substance abuse and the like which gives short-time relief; but the strategy itself begets further stress in future.

Adequate coping with stress, thus, is not only costly, but complex too. It requires attention, patience, accurate monitoring and execution of well-planned efforts.

Emotional predictors of coping : positive aspects

Egostrength : Self-reliance and dependability, self-trust, and lack of impulsivity, act as important stress buffers. This can also help individuals to refrain taking avoidance coping resources, namely, use of alcohol, smoke in excess (Friedman, Tucker, Schwartz, *et al*, 1995).

Self-esteem : Adequate self-esteem helps to moderate stress-relationship (Whisman & Know, 1993). High self-esteem can prove one's worth adequately and thereby affects the biophysiological functions of the individuals, viz., low-level of cortisol and ACTH in response to a challenging task (Seeman *et al*, 1995).

Self-image : Positive self-image provides strong determination, perseverance, less distractability, quick selection of right direction and timely execution to combat with stress. Self-confident and easy-going individuals, unlike highstrung individuals, cope with stressful events more effectively.

All the above qualities provide a meaning to one's life, the individual becomes definitely goal-oriented, scrupulous. Also, religious belief acts as an internal resource and helps to promote effective coping.

Adequate Arousability : This provides a capacity to re-set one's physiological arousal to pre-stress level at the earliest. Individuals with adequate stress modulation capacity, i.e., those with low Trait Anxiety, lower sensitivity to criticisms (can resist emotional disturbance) and social hassles, and with lower apprehension of some unpredicted doom, can maintain better and desired physiological homeostasis during stress. Capacity to re-set physiological level of arousal within a short-while is interlinked with one's biopsychosocial route of the organism. Moderate arousability can be evidenced through lower levels of catecholamines, corticosteroid, on the biochemical parameters, and on the physiological parameters through desired level of heart rate, blood pressure, pulse rate, pulse volume, skin conductance and so on.

Emotional predictors of coping : negative aspects

Inability to take responsibilities : Though a cross-section of the workers enjoy taking responsibilities, some shrink, for the latter, inability to exert control over job, causes stress. Lack of self-confidence vis-a-vis lack of control over job can cause deleterious effects onto the worker's physical and mental health (Bosma *et al*, 1997). They feel incompetent to tackle problems related to work environment also.

Feeling of inadequacy and inferiority : These personality characteristics cause excessive occupational stress. Reasons for developing such characteristics of personality have been detailed in this book. Such workers due to their feeling of ineptness perceive inadequacy over career development too. At times they don't opt for promotion, because promotion in service causes distress in them instead of happiness. Of course, the contrary is also true for some other workers who have feelings of adequacy and self-confidence. For the latter group, delayed promotion, insecurity over future job prospects cause psychological distress. Such distress can be taken as illness precursors.

(ii) **Inability to develop satisfying social relationship :** Poor social relationships with the supervisors—particularly with the colleagues and co-workers—causes job stress which in turn acts upon our health. For example, such job stress increases catecholamines and blood pressure and also increases the risk for heart disease (Davis *et al*, 1995). Mentally, it causes anxiety, depression, fear, and related other psychiatric symptoms. Interestingly, research reports suggest that work over-load could not be tied up with high blood pressure and other physical ailments when supportive relationship with office colleagues is maintained well. Therefore, social support helps both to combat stress and also to act as stress buffer in job stress.

(iii) **Role Playing :** Every individual, man or woman, has certain specific roles to play, though there may be some cultural variations. In Indian scenario, traditional female role consists of two major expectations—marriage mandate and motherhood mandate, whilst, for the males—it has primarily job mandate. The contemporary Indian scenario has changed, where women are getting engaged in career development and outside-family work. Be it whatever it may be, adequate role playing capacity develops out of parenting nurturing one has received since childhood, particularly during adolescence and early adulthood. If an individual, e.g., experiences difficulties in expressing disagreement, and goes to excessive extent of obtaining nurturance and support from others, he/she is likely to feel uncomfortable, helpless, and would develop insecurity in situations which demand self initiation of work. For example, initiation of a project in a work situation (Scully, 1996), or any such other assignment in any sphere of his life. It causes severe distress in the individual. Such individuals are likely to complain frequently of problems in adjustment which originate from 'role-conflict' and 'role-ambiguity'. Of course, role-conflict and role-ambiguity are not that uncommon phenomena in our life. Individuals with adequate role playing capacity can sort out such problems easily and independently, whilst for those with inadequate role playing it causes emotional distress.

Lack of control over work, i.e., when a person is unsure about what is to be done about the work he/she is assigned to, and also lacks knowledge about the standard methods to be employed for successful completion of the work —that causes role ambiguity. Thus, high psychological demands on job with little decision latitude can cause job stress. For example, a software engineer having three years' work experience with a given organisation was transferred to another branch of the same organisation in a different state on promotion. On joining the post he had been experiencing severe distress and came for counselling assistance. On enquiry it was revealed that the client had no idea about the work he was assigned nor did he know the technology be employed to complete that particular project. As he reported, the project leader (PL) did not cooperate with him in providing him assistance in this regard. Such job ambiguity gradually lead to depression in him.

When a person receives contradictory information about the standard methods of the work assigned, that leads to role conflict. For example, as opposed to that of the traditional Indian women's role, contemporary women are opting for job and career and they face relatively more family conflicts than those of men. Though some of the Indian families apparently seem to be generous to allow their daughter-in-laws to jobs and careers, they have unexpressed expectation that their daughter-in-laws should also perform efficiently home-role as well—where expectations from their sons regarding performance of home role is relatively less. Such a conflicting role causes stress and stress related symptoms in working women. When pressure increases at work both male and female report more conflicts due to their multiple commitments (Crouter *et al*, 1999).

Role conflict and role ambiguity can cause harmful effects onto the organism in the form of heightened catecholamine secretion, elevated pulse, blood pressure and such other symptoms. Pickering *et al*, (1996) found that, as a consequence of this job dissatisfaction, absenteeism, headache, high blood pressure, gastrointestinal and coronary diseases occur.

Recruitment/Job Placement and Stress—While selecting a job or assigning it, the worker and the employer should see that the nature of the work as well as the demands on the work must match well with the knowledge, abilities, and execution capacities of the employee so that the worker can excel his potentialities with maximum satisfaction. Also, the nature of the work be where the employee gets opportunity to exercise his choice or control at least to a certain extent—consequently he feels self-confident and better motivated to develop a challenging attitude within—to solve the problems. These are likely to lessen experience of stress.

(c) Work-family interface

Work-place stress via-a-vis family attitude as a source of stress—Work place stress can have deleterious effects on both the physical and mental health of the associates directly, and indirectly it causes serious problems in the family members of those associates. Stress at work can have substantial negative impact on the family and marital interaction (Perry *et al,* 2001). Contemporary workers experience work-family conflict which make them feel being pulled in multiple directions, i.e., demands from the work organisation and from the family.

Normally, family must not be viewed as a source of stress; rather, family be regarded as a major source to combat with stress, and family resources can buffer well against the adverse effects of stress. Family stress occurs when one attempts to combine multiple roles simultaneously. Mostly family stress is experienced by those who suffer from role conflict. For example, a worker—fails to perform his role as a husband, or as a father in the family. From this point of view the problem is more acute for women as people expect from the women to perform both the home role and the occupational-role simultaneously and equally well. Concessions to working parents, particularly working mothers in Indian families, are rarely made and, as such, conflict occurs between homemaker roles (household works, childcare, etc.) and work role (attending night shift, extra time to spend at office beyond duty schedule for attending emergency, for example, female doctors attending emergency O.T.) which enhances stress. Of course, women who have enough help and other resources, like, having some helping hand with the household works and child care, getting consent and cooperation from the husband and in-laws for continuing work, then that might be beneficial for women's overall well-being (feeling of self-sufficiency, better self-esteem and better life satisfaction) which can even lower health hazards, namely, coronary risk (Weidner *et al,* 1997). It does not mean that men are not distressed owing to role conflict. Multiple role can take their toll on men as well, though men and women are distressed because of different kinds of events, for example, the former are more stressed by financial constraints. Usually work overload refrains men from adequate interaction with family members—particularly with their children. Such parents get easily distressed owing to varieties of problems their children complain of, for example, those related to their academic issues and social interaction. However, marriage is protective for men and women —both with respect to their physical and mental health (Rushing, Ritter & Burton, 1992).

Despite negative effects of role conflict and role overload, there may be some positive effects also of such conflicts which arise out of home-and-work responsibilities. If an individual takes it positively, then combining motherhood and other home role with that of employment role can be beneficial for improving her self-esteem and self-satisfaction. Consideration of role-conflict and role-overload positively depends on the one hand upon the attitude and perception of the individuals, and, on the other, social support, particularly family supports he/she received. Family attitude, if it constantly creates a negative force, becomes more distressing for both men and women.

Through stress management training one can learn to cope with multiple roles—then it can buffer one against health problems and can enhance one's self-esteem and general well-being.

2. The Work and the Work Environment

(a) **Work Environment (Physical environment)**—Work place which does not provide sufficient light and air-circulation and suitable temperature (Leka & Griffiths, 2005) such a stuffy and polluted physical envorenment is stressful. Similarly works which demand regular exposure as a matter of course to physical and chemical hazards, can cause serious biological injuries. For example, constant exposure to noise, radiation, and the like can cause respiratory and cardiovascular diseases and even cancer. According to WHO (1996), health does not mean mere absence of disease or sickness, but a positive state of complete physical, mental and social well-being. A work environment which doesn't foster stress is one which not only takes appropriate steps to control harmful environmental conditions to which workers are exposed, but provides abundance of health (Leka & Griffiths, 2005) promoting opportunities too for the workers.

(b) **Ergonomics and Environmental design**—Modern equipments be used and employees be provided with facilities to update their expertise to keep pace with the modernisation of equipments. It reduces hazards related to design and management of work. It can minimise imbalance between work pressure and resources of the employee. Risk management factors have been delineated by Leka & Griffiths (2005) in this context. For example, work-pressure but fewer resources, namely, instrumental facilities, lack of adequate manpower, add a psychological sense of overload (Nowack & Wimer, 2011). If risk factors of work can be controlled well and work environment is healthy, this can make work itself self-promoting.

(c) **Work pressure**—The employer demands time bound work and creates pressure on the employee with very little concern (Leka & Griffiths, 2005) about the employees' knowledge and expertise, work environment and available facilities. Moderate to high degree of work pressure over a period of long time doesn't allow one to find time for recreation. The workers sometimes even fail to enjoy scheduled holidays. At times, some workers are to remain constantly alert even when they are away from their respective work place. They remain engaged throughout on internet, laptop and similar other electronic mediums for online management of work-related problems. For example, in India, in corporate organisations, when employee has to be in touch with a client who is in America or in England, for example, he may have to sacrifice night sleep to continue online discussion adjusting time variations between the two countries, and so on. Consequently, in recent years, high-job stress has been found to be associated with health-risk, namely, coronary heart diseases (Davis, Matthews, Meilahn & Kiss, 1995). Young associates within 35-45 years of age are recently found to be at high-risk for coronary heart problems than their senior associates.

This of course must not mean that stress occurs only when the demand and pressure of work exceed the worker's ability to cope with. Stress also is equally experienced by a worker when his knowledge and expertise are not sufficiently utilised, evaluated, and reinforced by the organisations. Therefore, it must not mean as an axiom that work load and work pressure always cause stress; rather very low work pressure to the extent that the employee fails to exert his efficiencies sufficiently creates equal stressful experience to the employee.

Actually work-pressure is unavoidable, especially in the recent era, due to high competitive work culture. One cannot totally avoid it, but one has to learn how to tackle it without stress. It depends upon the personality characteristics and available resources and attitude of the worker. Pressure of work may not always be perceived negatively. In fact, pressure can create a challenging attitude in the worker which keeps him alert, well-motivated to learn techniques to handle the problems efficiently. However, if a given worker perceives pressure as unmanageable and excessive—to that extent that it makes him feel helpless and exhausted—that stress is harmful both to the individual's health as well as to the organisation's progress. A healthy job means that the pressures created on the employees are appropriate to the abilities and resources of the employees so that they can complete the work with full confidence and remain satisfied.

(d) **Shifting duty**—Poorer physical and mental functioning have been associated with job hours, travelling schedule, rotating shifts, and, especially, night shifts. Due to inadequate sleep, fatigue sets in which can lead to poor performance and even accidents—particularly for those who work with instruments (Nowack & Wimer, 2011).

(e) **The work**—Job must not go against the workers' values. Not only that, hours of job, sudden/frequent travelling schedule, rotating shifts, heavy demands to complete work on deadline of submission cause stress, one has to look into the fact that it is also equally distressing (Nowack & Wimer, 2011) if workers fail to maintain their values in work situation. But in developing countries like India, many a times situation demands that owing to financial constraints one gets enrolled with a job which is against his social status. In such cases many workers present a false self to the society, which is harmful to his mental and physical health. However, congenial work environment and cooperation amongst workers sometimes help to overcome such stress at least temporarily. Particularly blue collar jobs, compared to white- and pink-collar jobs, are more stress-producing and injurious to physical and mental health (Nowack & Wimer, 2011). Employer's support and sympathetic attitude toward workers can help to combat such self-distressing experience in the employees.

(f) **Frequent change in the nature of the job assigned and also sudden shift from one group to the other with whom to work**—Workers, especially the juniors, feel stressed due to frequent change in the nature of the work. Such a change also alters the work environment. i.e., the boss and the colleagues to work with. This weakens group morale. Frequent and sudden change cause confusion in the employees as they feel less competent to keep pace with such change. In some organisations, when a given project is complete, some of the associates remain unassigned for quite some time. Such a vacuum feeling bring negative impression about the management.

It results in severe aggression, worries and frustration in the workers and kills motivation for work. This causes frequent absenteeism and tendency to change work organisations. In Robinson & Morrison's (1995) term, in such situations the employee lacks 'citizenship behaviour' towards the organisation. On the one hand, constant anxiety that prevails in the workers over economic recovery of the organisation and continuing thread of downsizing, on the other lack of information to the workers about impending restructuring creates 'panic' (Nowack & Wimer, 2011) in them.

(g) **Work overload**—This is another source of occupational stress. Workers who require to be involved in multinature works, also to deal with too hard works and that too with notorious irregular duty roster—feel more stressed. On the one hand work overload and on the other lack of time to care for their health, also for interaction with their family members, and lack of vacations make them more vulnerable to high risk for illness, namely, diabetes, high blood pressure, gastric ulcer and coronary heart disease (Davis *et al*, 1995). What is most important in this context is the perception of work overload by a given worker. The latter shows a consistent relationship between experience of stress and related physical illness. How variability issues in perception can occur due to psychological get-up of an individual has been detailed in the section on personality characteristics and work stress.

(h) **Financial packages and other facilities provided**—It doesn't require special mention that the financial reward and/or salary package is the best rewarding agent to any worker. Sometimes workers are ready to compromise with low salary if many ancillary facilities are provided to them. Management must not fail to keep commitment in this respect. Sudden recess in the financial package is highly stressful to any worker. Psychologically it demoralises the worker as they consider it as a violation of contract. Violation of contract can lead to resentment and lower level of commitment to organisation (Rousseau, 2004 and Nowack & Wimer, 2011). Perhaps it would be better to see that pay will be contingent upon one's performance. This can avoid the problem of over-paid—which is no less stressful than that of unpaid or low paid (Nowack & Wimer, 2011).

(i) **Technostress**—Rapid progress in techno world had made our life simpler. We can solve our regular life hassles easily and quickly, yet sometimes we turnout to be its victims and suffer from its adverse consequences. For example, it increases productivity enormously but in turn, creates excessive pressure and work-load onto the employees on whom the annual turnover of the organisation depends. Such constant pressure has insidious deterimental effects on one's physical and mental health. From this sense, techno-resource has been designated as 'double-edged sword' by Nowack & Wimer (2011). Parallel to that of productivity, it has virtually snatched time from many executives to relax and enjoy time with their family members. Even when on holidays, many executives practically spend their entire vacation responding to their e-mails, voice mails, and sometimes they become compelled to rush to their work place leaving the entire family in a sort of distress. This contributes to the "let-down effects" (Nowack & Wimer, 2011) and makes them sick.

(j) **Other factors**—Perceived inequalities in promotion vis-a-vis perceived inadequate carrier prospects, perceived insecurity over job prospect, and uncertainty over continuity of job (sudden downsizing, sudden reduction in pay packages, Nowack & Wimer, 2011) or causal and temporary employment can cause job stress which finally leads to anxiety, depression and many other forms of psychological distress (Reynolds, 1997).

Chapter 3

BEHAVIOURAL AND HEALTH SIGNS OF STRESS RELATED DISORDERS

Home life—its complexities, competitions, jealousies, frustrations, and boredom as well as working conditions which involve one into a perpetual striving for security related to his achievement, prestige, or drives for comradeship in relation to colleagues and authority are common stressful problems in our lives. Personal interaction that gives rise to anxiety, hostility, aggression, guilt, bottled-up resentment and discontent may act as the cause for the manifestation of somatic ill-health, popularly known as psychosomatic symptoms which is recently designated as psychophysiological symptoms.

Prolonged tension and anxiety not only besets human psyche, it upsets his physiology as well. Though physical symptoms in such disorders dominate the clinical picture, their mental genesis—the meaning to the symptom, that an individual attributes, are not superficially recognisable. Frequently, the manifestations of symptoms in such disorders are determined more by personality characteristics than by the nature of the etiological agents which produce the symptoms. It is therefore, not only that illness in itself is important for treatment, but also that particular meaning which has been attributed to a particular symptom by a given patient is equally important. However, for easy understanding, the dysfunctions usually reported may briefly be narrated considering the various physical symptoms involves.

Some commonly reported physical illnesses related to stress are :

Cardiovascular System

Stress inducing emotional change contributes to the development of coronary artery disease, angina pectoris, and myocardial infarction and the like in various forms of heart failure. Constant exposure to stress causes high blood pressure. High blood pressure creates undue pressure on the blood vessel walls, which may burst and cause a stroke. It also over-pressures the circulatory system and puts excessive strain on the heart, which in turn may lead to heart attacks. These conditions are determined by multiple factors—genetic and constitutional—which are reflected in biochemical predispositions, namely, lipid metabolism. The latter is modifiable through experience of stress, e.g., fear and anxiety.

Hypertension

Vascular hypertension is considered a systemic reaction rather than a specific disease. Inner tension, suppressed and repressed emotion inadequately discharged either verbally or through physical activities, excessive rage is manifested in hypertension. Awareness of this disease may cause apprehension of other related physical ailments like, high blood pressure, and gastrointestinal problems in some cases.

High blood pressure

It has just been narrated that constant exposure to stress, and related apprehension cause high blood pressure.

Muscle aches and pain

Migraine

It is episodic and usually unilateral headache. This is splitting and throbbing in nature occurs periodically and usually after period of tension. Predominantly there is a neurovascular dysfunction with associated physical symptoms and low mood. Sufferers of migraine are usually of perfectionistic personality. They attach great significance to life achievement and require their family members also to conform to the same. Family environment usually restricts free expression of aggression which, in turn, causes heightened arousal and suppressed rage and hostility. The latter condition precipitates such reaction. Sibling rivalries, hostility towards family members, for example, are reported by such patients during psychotherapeutic sessions.

Tension Headache

This occurs due to prolonged and sustained contracture of the cervical musculature produced out of chronic anxiety (Chattopadhyay, Majumder & Basu, 1982; Chattopadhyay & Majumder, 1982), severe tension, feeling of insecurity, inferiority, conflicts of various types and rigidity and certain obsessional personality characteristics. Contraction of cervical musculature produces diffused and sustained aching pain in the forehead, back of the head, shoulders and neck of the sufferers. Executives who constantly watch clock and sit dissatisfied at their desks are the victims of tension headache. Also, fast tempo of modern life, lack of relaxation, non-cooperative family environment can be responsible for tension headache. Relief of anxiety helps them to get rid of it.

Torticollis (functional) and other psychological pain syndrome (psychalgia)

Tightness in our muscles occurs during period of stress (Sanyal, Chattopadhyay & Biswas, 1998). This causes disorder of the movement of the posture of the head and neck, often associated with neck muscles and forehead muscles. In case of torticollis functional, though no organic basis is evident through X-ray etc., the patient complains of muscle spasms and both atrophy and hypertrophy of neck muscles (Mukhopadhyay, Basu & Chattopadhyay, 1994). Muscle contraction also causes Writers' cramp and backache, in some cases.

The term 'psychalgia' refers to pain of a psychological origin (Raber, 1985), i.e., when pain occurs without any detectable organic dysfunction behind it. Author's personal research in this area showed that (Chattopadhyay, Bhaduri, Basu & Basu, 1990) in case of the patients with organic dysfunction, X-ray report and other examinations revealed a positive finding of identifiable tissue damage, whereas, in case of the patients with functional pain (psychalgia), though are similar intractable low back-pain, neck pain like that of the organic group was noted, but no radiological and other necessary supports for the same were evident. Also, the latter group of patients, on various psychological tests, obtained significantly higher scores on neuroticism, anxiety, guilt, hopelessness, helplesseness, internal aggression, depression, and tendency to suppress their emotional conflicts in comparison to the patients with organic pain syndrome. Therefore, personality predisposition of the patients seem to responsible for manifestation of psychalgia. Patients with psychalgia often cause failure in their management by their physicians and this has intrigued medical practitioners to urge for research with a view to look into the psychological factors involved in psychalgia.

Backache

About 80% of the ache at the back of the neck and shoulder and low back ache is due to tension we face in the modern competitive society. Some of the executives report backache when they face problems. Tension causes contraction of the muscles. Once worry is over, the muscles gradually relax and body aches disappear. Individual differences in perception of stress and selection of coping strategy (Chatterjee, 2008), and personality characteristics of the sufferers have been reported significant (Chatterjee, 2004) in understanding etiology of the patients with functional neck pain and low-back pain.

Gastrointestinal System

Peptic Ulcer

It may occur under a number of circumstances. Psychologically, any conflict inducing anxiety and worries lead to gastric hyperactivity and prolonged hydrochloric acid (HCI) secretion causes ulceration. These individuals usually remain dissatisfied in their life—may be in the domain of life achievement, or in family and social interaction. From psychoanalytic point of view such patients are found to have a persisting strong infantile wish to be loved and cared for. Essentially they possess infantile personality with extreme dependency longings. Some of them report threatful experience in the sexual functioning—threat may be in reality or in fantasy. Their life conflicts are often heightened by external circumstances which induce stressful anxiety in them. It is known that anxiety and aggressive strivings increase motility, vascularity, secretion and electrical activity of the stomach. The reverse is applicable in relation to functions of the stomach in depression. Excessive stomach acid during stress may be excreted that can destroy the stomach walls and proliferation of stomach cells occur. Also, stress tenses and contracts the muscles of the stomach and thus prevents proper digestion of food.

Alimentary System

Mucus Colitis

Though the prime symptom is constipation and discharge of mucus-containing stools, anxiety producing symptoms are found to be associated with it. The patient complaints are of indigestion and irregular appetite. The patient with a view to avoid discomfort resorts to an increasing restriction of diet. Anxiety-related symptoms like distension of the stomach, belching, flatulence, nausea, and gastric symptoms are present. Mostly patients are of asthenic bodybuilt. In a good number of cases this physiological disturbance appears to be in response to anxiety, fear, guilt, high sensitivity, overconsciousness and resentment.

Ulcerative Colitis

The onset and exacerbation of this symptom has been frequently associated with a sudden unforeseen threat to the patient's security. Threat may be at the personal level, namely amputation or loss at career achievement, or else death, separation, rejection and some such other events in the family. These patients react to loss with depression and rage, accompanied by disorganisation of bowel function. Life history of such patients usually reveal helpless infancy, need for protective care from mother at the childhood, but mother turned out to be hostile and rejecting. Since childhood, hostility is found to have been ingrained in them, but due to dependency need they fail to be hostile. Any expression of rage gives them a feeling of guilt and fear of retaliation, which makes them further apprehensive and insecured. Emotionally, they seem to have impaired capacity for appropriate affective experiences, yet they are, in actuality, found to be perceptive and sensitive to the emotional responsiveness of others. Thus, they are ambivalent in interaction style. Intensive dynamic psychotherapy helps them to manage their discomfort.

Irritable Bowel Syndrome (IBS)

There are many underlying causes of IBS but stress undoubtedly plays an important part in it. Stress research shows that the patient with IBS improves when they are removed from the stress factors.

Musculoskeletal system

Rheumatoid arthritis

Emotional stress, for example, threat of loss of important figures in life, disappointment in the personal relations of the patients precipitate the onset and exacerbation of this illness. These patients are found to be composed emotionally, prefer to swallow emotional reactions to others, rather than its over-expression. Domineering mother induces fear in the child and thereby dependency on others is masked. Feelings of resentment, rebellion, and hostility with associated guilt are present in them. Control of intense hostility is accomplished through neuromuscular activity. Perhaps it provides a satisfaction through control over the environment. Rheumatoid arthritis results from a disorder on the immune system of the body. Stress affects the immune system and, as such, aggravates the severity of the arthritis.

Respiratory system

Asthma

Since the time of Hippocrates an association has been found to exist between emotional arousal and asthmatic attack. Despite the fact that asthma occurs in individuals with a constitutional predisposition, there are many cases in which the attacks are initiated by events other than the presence of a specific antigen. Hyperventilation leads to bronchial spasm, its precipitation through induction of anxiety may also be causative in initiation of the asthmatic episode. A relationship between asthmatic attack and arousal due to repressed psychological conflicts has been recorded. Personality characteristics and nature of psychosexual development also have been considered while treating such patients.

Endocrine-Metabolic Systems

Diabetes

The most common types of diabetes are insulin-dependent diabetes mellitus (Type I), and non-insulin dependent diabetes mellitus (Type II). The latter has been associated with emotional stress, while the former is sometimes found to have juvenile onset which is insidious in nature. Urinary and blood glucose levels are elevated following periods of emotional arousal, and the glucose tolerance curves may be modified at such times. In general, the glucose-tolerance test has been found to indicate a higher degree of diabetes when the individual feels more hostile and depressed, while the reverse is true when the patient feels relaxed and cared for.

Thyroid dysfunctions

Malfunctioning of thyroid glands can result not only from physical causes but from psychological stress as well.

Menstrual disturbances

Three types of such disturbances have been connected with psychological and emotional factors : (i) amenorrhoea, (ii) premenstrual or menstrual tension, and (iii) dysmenorrhoea. Amenorrhoea is an abnormal suppression or absence of menstrual flow. Emotional factors can cause a temporary delay in the onset of menstrual flow. A somewhat rare instance of the phenomenon is called 'pseudocyesis' (fasle pregnancy). It is, of course, an extreme form of amenorrhoea in that it involves a total psychopathology rather than just an isolated symptom.

Women who experience premenstrual-menstrual pain and tension are mostly found to be moody, easily irritable and sufferers of severe anxiety. Personality types frequently associated with this disorder are those of women who rebel against their femininity. They show very defensive personality. Mostly their sexual and maternal functions have been reported to be frustrated. They are mostly aggressive, assertive and competitive with men (Chattopadhyay & Das, 1980).

Dysmenorrhoea is difficult or painful menstruation. This is commonly accompanied by symptoms such as tension, anxiety, fatigue, headache, and insomnia.

Menopause

Menopausal symptoms represent a complex of physiological and psychological responses to which the mature women usually adopt more effectively than those who have neurotic or psychotic personality characteristics. More disturbances are noted in those women who are anxious, agitated and have tendency to exaggerate.

Likewise, impotencies in men, frigidity in women and infertility have been associated with psychological and emotional factors (Mukhopadhyay & Chattopadhyay, 1994). When it is evident that emotional factors are the primary causes for determining the existence of these conditions, depth psychotherapy is the indicated treatment.

Libidinal dysfunctions

Diminished and/or failure to perform adequate sexual functions have been associated with experience of stress. Feelings of shame, disgust, guilt, fear and hatred also are found responsible for it. In men, the common psychosomatic symptoms are impotencey and premature ejaculation. Frigidity, dysmenorrhoea, amenorrhoea, premenstrual tensions are common expressions in women. In both the sexes, infertility has been recently associated with stress; this is called psychogenic infertility/idiopathic infertility (Mukhopadhyay & Chattopadhyay, 1994).

Predominantly, metabolic dysfunctions are—

Obesity

Sometimes people under stress tend to indulge in excessive eating. Frequent eating provides a sort of comfort to them. Comfort in the sense that being engaged in eating they make them able to enjoy for a while which serves to relieve them of stress and they can relax at least for a while. Therefore, frequent eating and in some cases excessive eating results in weight gain. This, is turn, is likely to cause physical illnesses like heart problem, diabetes, arthritis, and so on.

As opposed to 'development obesity', Brush (cited by Kolb, 1973) has coined the term 'reactive obesity' to separate out those problems of overweight that occur suddenly after a psychologically traumatic incidence in persons who have not been evidenly stout previously. History shows that previously they used to react to stress with overating. Personality characteristics and family patterns are very similar to those with 'developmental obesity'.

Anorexia Nervosa

This is a somewhat uncommon psychophysiological reaction. For a sizeable patient group with this disorder the primary concern is not phobic avoidance of food, per se. They indulge in episodic gorging with food, coupled later with guilt and induction of vomiting. In another smaller group the primary drive in phobic avoidance of food and eating, per se, because taking in food has symbolic representation to them, like disgust, impregnation, or some such other meaning. This reaction occurs largely in young single woman. They are mostly intellectually superior but in personality they are introverted, stubborn, selfish, perfectionistic, overtly sensitive, compulsive and self-punitive in nature.

Skin (Dermatitis)

Skin is a good index of emotion. Because its surface is supplied by a multitude of small blood vessels that are under the control of the autonomic nervous system. Common skin disorders which are caused or aggravated by emotional arousal are neurodermatitis, eczema, and itching.

Alpoecia areata

Excessive hair loss. This condition has been described where emotional factors play important role. Small patches of hair from a circumscribed area of head starts falling.

Trichotolomania

Patients complain of a compulsive urge to pull hair of the head, so much so that the patients end-up to be bald-headed and requires to use wig while meeting public. Pulling hair doesn't cause any pain to the patient. He becomes victim of a bad habit due to excessive tension and anxiety.

Others

Insomnia and Fatigue

The release of stress hormone under influence of stress stimulates the brain preparing it to respond to the external stressor. Under constant or prolonged stress, the elevated level of stress hormones tend to keep the brain in an alert state and this causes the person to have difficulty going to sleep. When insomnia continues for a prolonged period, the person gets exhausted—leading ultimately to chronic fatigue.

Cancer

It is believed that stress is a major factor which causes many different types of cancer. The reason being that stress weakens the immune system, which makes our body more susceptible to the "invasion" by cancer cells (particularly NK cells) (Bandyopadhyay, Chattopadhyay, Ghosh *et al*, 1987; Chattopadhyay, Bandyopadhyay, Basu *et al*, 1989).

Chapter 4

INTERVENTION : SOME SPECIFIC TECHNIQUES

Intervention strategy may be applied either in individual set-up, namely one-to-one psychotherapeutic/counselling sessions, or in group set-up, namely, workshop programmes offered at workplace. Both the set-ups have their own merits and demerits. When workers complain of certain physical illnesses, like, tension, tensionheadache, high blood pressure, obesity, irritable bowel syndrome, alcohol/drug abuse, or individuals with cardiovascular diseases, e.g., angina or myocardial infarction, and those with psychological problems, like personality inadequacy, inferiority, work or any other situation/event/person related phobia, anxiety, or low mood due to personal and emotional problems, they are often trained with coping strategies in individual one-to-one sessions. Of late, certain intervention strategies are being offered in group set-up at work place itself for workers who complain of some general sources of stress, namely techno stress.

Though some of the sources of stress can be traced back to individual factors, viz, personality characteristics, coping strategies, there are also many organisational sources of stress. Without addressing organisational sources of stress, individual stress management programme for work stress is likely to be ineffective (Nowack & Wimer, 2011). Organisational sources of stress and work as a source of stress have been delineated separately in Chapter 2. Let us examine now some of the possible methods of intervention which could be lateral to the sources of stress mentioned so far. Intervention techniques which could be implemented from the organisational perspective have been narrated in chapter 19— 'Prevention of Stress'. Intervention techniques applicable to workers will now be described briefly.

Methods generally employed for management of stress present a wide array of psychological techniques. Whatever it may be while applying any techniques for any stress management programme the resource person has to make sure that the individual, at the very outset of the programme, understands well (a) what stress is, (b) how to identify stressors and (c) stressors can create physical wear and tear. Once the participant(s) has (have) learnt these then in the second stage, he/they can be taught about certain techniques for practice and self-help. Final stage is the stage of application of these techniques. To start with it is desired that the individual applies a given technique under supervision and later can apply on himself under self-supervision, provided be is certified by the counsellor about self-administration of the technique. Prior to application of a given technique, goal setting is essential for every individual under stress and thus techniques would vary from man to man and time onwards, depending upon individual variations in goal setting, i.e., setting of target behaviour for amelioration of stress.

A wide array of cognitive-behavioural therapy techniques have been employed so far to combat stress. To name some of these—self-monitoring, modification of internal dialogue, positive self-talk, self-instruction, contingency contracting, and stress inoculation programme.

Some of the techniques employed for group training programmes will now be described briefly.

Behavioural Techniques

Behavioural techniques include biofeedback, progressive muscular relaxation (PMR) training and meditation.

In PMR, the client under supervision is taught to relax his entire body following certain steps. Initially, the client is requested to lie down or to sit in a recliner, for a couple of minutes with eyes closed in a semi-dark and sound-proof room till he experiences reduced muscle tone. Then, the client is taught, purposefully, to tense and then to relax each body part separately with the goal to gain introspective feeling of relief from tension through auto-control. For example, the client is instructed to clench his right fist first, and then slowly to tighten it up to its maximum (for 10 seconds) then gradually to release till it reaches a placid state and maintain the position for about 20 seconds. The time estimation should be approximate without any counting, consultation or referring the clock. Similar procedure to be followed for the left fist, and, then, both fists together. Thereafter, the process is to be followed for all his body parts from forehead to toe (initially under supervision, till the supervisor certifies him to continue the procedure by himself). The order of muscle group to be focussed on—the standard procedure has been described by Jacobson (1983). Since the process is gradual hence the nosology "Progressive Muscle Relaxation" (Jacobson, 1938). Tensing (activation of sympathetic division of the ANS), and relaxation (activation of parasympatheric division of the ANS) of the muscles are done alternatively with a view to bring a balance between the functions of the sympathetic and parasympathetic parts of the ANS. Needless to mention that, for the high-stressed individuals, sympathetic division of the ANS mostly remains at higher level, which make them high strung.

In PMR all the body parts are involved, viz., face, neck, shoulder arms, stomach, thigh angles and feet preceded and followed by whole body relaxation called '*Shabasana*'. According to Patanjali (Prasad, 1982) of the eight systems of yoga, posture *(asanas)*, breath regulating exercise (pranayama), and meditation *(dhyana)* are most important in the management of stress disorder (Udupa, 1985). Combinaion of yogic techniques (Sridhar, 1981) and yogic relaxation and biofeedback together showed reduction in blood pressure in hypertension disorder and many other psychosomatic disorders (Vahia, Doongaji, Jeste *et al*, 1973).

Another important technique is training of time management. For the clients/ associates who are predisposed to high stress (owing to their personal appraisal of life situations/events) always perceive high pressure of work, and stress is produced by the feeling that they have too many things to do, but apprehension of whether would be able to complete each one perfectly and within deadline. They usually lack time-management skills. Time management programme includes (Heeker & Thorpe, 2005) the following steps : (i) specific goals for works, (ii) priorising one's goals, (iii) to eliminate activities that consume time with little pay-off, and (iv) setting aside specific blocks for specific activities.

In problem-solving training (Heeker & Thorpe, 2005) the associates are helped to learn first—to define a given problem. Then they should learn to generate means for solution of the problems. These should be generated depending upon the available resources they have within their access. Thirdly, they are to be helped to implement the same selected and finally to reevaluate the outcome based on the solution means chosen.

Cognitive behaviour therapy (CBT) is important for life stress management. Also Beck's cognitive therapy (Beck & Weishar, 1995), Ellis's rational emotive behaviour therapy (REBT) (Ellis, 1995), and strees inoculation training (Meichenbaum & Turk, 1982) all have been used in stress management. Basic theoretical background and methods of all these have been discussed in chapters 4 and 5 of this book.

In addition to the above mentioned therapeutic strategies, self-control techniques (Heeker & Thorpe, 2005) and social support are used as stress moderators to help clients learn self-managements of stress. Individuals with a strong sense of personal control experience less stress in response to stressors than those with a poorer sense of self-control (Sarafino, 1994; cited by Heeker & Thorpe, 2005). Therapists help the clients recognise which aspects of their lives they can control better and to obtain mastery over that. This can be done through—

(a) Identification of what can make one-self truly absorbed (except substance abuse) when he wants to cut him off of the work situation.

(b) This provides him mental relief. It is further better to build habit of regular involvement in some physical exercise like walking, jogging, relaxation which will make him feel physically fit and energetic.

Development of 'positivistic life style' also includes food habit—regular intake of balance diet, and restful sleep.

(c) To accept that in the present era life means stress. Instead of avoiding stress and imagining/expecting/wishing a total stress-free life, it would be better to select strategies to face life stress, at least those which are inevitable.

Likewise, clients are encouraged and taught to develop and maintain supportive relationship so that social-support can buffer life stress.

Another approach to relaxation, viz., meditation is also used by clinicians for inducing relaxation and reducing physiological arousal (Smith, Hocksena *et al*, 2003). Meditation, on the one hand, helps to control distracting thoughts progressively and finally to reach a state of deep concentration (when the individual is free from unwanted distracting thoughts related to materialistic world), and, on the other, indirectly brings the body in a totally resting condition. Meditation beings a significant lowering of the respiratory rate and heart-rate, stabilizes blood pressure and brings the EEG brain waves too suggesting decreased cortical arousal (Smith, Hocksena *et al*, 2003). Meditation has been proved effective in reducing symptoms of depression, chronic anxiety, excessive anger, cardio-pulmonary and gastrointestinal symptoms (Speca, Carlson, Goodey & Angen, 2000), and also in reducing tension headache

(Vasudevan, Kumaraih, Mishra & Balodhi, 1994), and relapse in people prone to serious depression (Snaith, 1998). Psychologically, meditation brings greater concentration, stable temperament, and enhanced self-esteem.

Biofeedback

The term 'biofeedback' was coined in the late 1960s to describe laboratory procedures. Thereafter it has been being used to train experimental research subjects to alter brain activity, blood pressure, heart rate, and other bodily functions that normally cannot be controlled voluntarily. It is based on the theory that stressful events produce strong emotions, which arouse certain physical responses. Many of these responses are controlled by the sympathetic nervous system, the network of nerve tissues that helps prepare the body to meet emergency situations.

In behavioural medicine, learning principles are applied to modify one's physiological processes. The principles are drawn from operant and classical conditioning. It is based on the assumptions that learning principles have significant role to play in the development, maintenance, and treatment of physical illnesses. Therefore, while applying techniques which are based on learning principles, it is thought that, individuals can be helped to modify risk behaviour and manage negative emotions and thoughts which contribute to illness, though traditionally it used to be thought that modification of one's own physiological processes (covert behaviour) are not under the individual's direct voluntary control.

Biofeedback refers to a set of techniques which enables the individual to employ auto-control even if external stress inducing stimulus is present (Mukhopadhyay, Basu & Chattopadhyay, 1994). In this, the individual is exposed to certain information regarding his internal physiological functions. Physiological functions are measured through different psychophysiological parameters and the individual is provided with those obtained information (data) through audio-visual devices using computer screen. The parameters are recorded using electrodes and selection of the parameters are done depending upon the symptoms (related target organ) the individual reports. For example, in case of tension headache, frontalies muscles are the target organs, whereas trapezious muscles are the target organs, in case of, for example, writers' cramp (Mukhopadhyay, Basu & Chattopadhyay, 1994). Measures used may be EMG (Kumaraih, 1980), EEG, skin conductance, blood pressure (Rau *et al*, 2003) and so on. This author used biofeedback method for treatment of subjects who suffered either from high or low blood pressure. Feedback from equipments measuring an index of the participant's blood pressure on each heart cycle was delivered to a computer screen so that growing green bars indicated changes in the right direction and growing red bars indicated changes in the wrong direction. In addition, verbal reinforcement like 'You did it the right way' also was provided. After 3 training sessions the participants were able to lower or raise their blood pressure. Those authors suggested that a course of biofeedback can be helpful to complement a drug regimen. Since information received about the internal physiological status of the individual are fed back to the individual to modify that state and to maintain equilibrium, hence the technique is called 'Biofeedback'.

Biofeedback training can be taken as an operant learning process. The feedback signal may also act as a kind of reward for reducing tension. Any successful learning requires reward. Biofeedback machine acts as a kind of 'sixth sense' (http://www.aapb.org) which allows patients to see or hear activity going on inside their bodies. For example, the machine used is competent to pick up electrical signals in the muscles. It translates these signals into a form that patients can detect. It triggers a flash light, bulb, or activates a beeper as and when muscles grow more tensed. The aim of the patient on biofeedback training is to relax tense muscles and thus they try to slow down the flushing or beeping signals. The biofeedback machine can detect a person's internal bodily functions with greater sensitivity and precision than a person can do alone through continuous feedback from the machine. For example, a given patient's heart rate might be converted into a tone, so that the patient can hear how fast or slowly his heart is beating. The patient efforts to change the bodily process. The patient learns what thoughts or behaviour will modify the bodily functions. For example, a patient might learn that blocking out all sounds, concentrating, and breathing slowly help to reduce heart rate (Taylor, 1994), However, exceptions are also reported.

For tension headache patients (Kumaraih, 1980) electrodes are attached to the forehead of the patient and muscle contractions are electronically detected, amplified, and feedback to the person either visually (through computer screen) or auditorily (through tone signal). The signal increases the pitch when the muscles contract and decreases when it relaxes. The client is trained to keep muscles relaxed following the tone signal. Likewise, for the clients with hypertension, the client's blood pressure is monitored. The client is rewarded by feedback in the form of tone or light signal when he succeeds in lowering blood pressure and can relax. Within 4-8 weeks time the clients learn to recognise the onset of tension and can reduce it at a desired level without receiving any feedback information from the machine (Thorpe & Olson, 1994; Mukhopadhyay & Turner, 1997). In our laboratory we have successfully treated chronic patients with muscular disorders (i.e., patients with functional torticolis, and finger jerking) within a short time applying biofeedback technique (Mukhopadhyay, Basu & Chottopadhyay, 1994). Patients usually are taught some form of relaxation exercise. Some patients learn to identify the circumstances that trigger their symptoms. They are also taught how to cope with stressful events. It helps in gaining patient's self-control.

Biofeedback is mostly applied on patients with migraine headache, tension headache, and many other types of pain, disorders of digestive system, high or low blood pressure, cardiac arrhythmias, Raynand's disease (a circulatory disorder that causes uncomfortably cold hands). Of late, it is used for patients with epilepsy, paralysis and other movement disorders (Runck, www.psychotherapy.com, 2011). Also patients with anxiety and those with functional torticolis (Mukhopadhyay, Basu & Chattopadhyay, 1994) show improvement after biofeedback treatment.

Biofeeback techniques are useful tools to help one learn to control his nervous system and achieve relaxation. The biofeedback information is valuable to direct progress of treatment also.

Comments

Some of the organisations prefer only work place workshops, like demonstrations to teach their workers intervention techniques, no matter whether that type of group demonstration, in actuality, helps each worker to solve his/her inner conflicts which cause stress in them. Such organisations think that individual sessions with workers will take away much of their working hours causing damage to the annual turnover of the organisation. In fact, such attitude of the organisations does not help to ameliorate stress on the workers who require personal attention, rather such attitude begets further stress in the workers finally causing damage to the annual work output. This very attitude of the organisations is not conductive to workstress management. Providing health scheme facilities to the workers must not be done in a matter-of-fact-way. This is not something to show other organisations that health scheme programmes are in vogue and practice. Such schemes must be implemented adequately. Otherwise, the work environment may be regarded as non-cooperative, indifferent, and non-productive (Leka & Griffiths, 2005) and stress-inducing. In such situations, not the workers, but the management personnel need to be exposed to awareness programme with a view to learn that until internal conflicts and stress-inducing sources are tapped individually in the workers, group demonstration will be of little worth. Factors like personality inadequacy, inferiority cannot be dealt with in group set-up. Moreover, without prior consent of the worker, his/her individual problems must not be disclosed and remedies must not be suggested publicly, which is unethical and can create medico-legal allegations against the counsellor in the long run.

Some of the techniques, viz., time-management training, training of assertiveness, confidence building, interpersonal interaction, and muscular relaxation may be demonstrated through work-place, workshop. Interestingly, in such work shop sessions, it is found that many of the workers personally meet the demonstrator and seek one-to-one sessions for discussing their personal matters cofidentially. Individual problems which are complex and can't be dealt with alone can be solved by taking counselling assistance from qualified clinical psychologists or counsellors (Leka & Griffiths, 2005). Organisations should take feedback from such specialists later to provide adequate facilities to the distressed workers. Contemporary organisations are expected to change their traditional conservative outlook and. not to be totally work-oriented only ignoring human factors. Basic requirements for implementing health; promotion schemes in work place is to make the work culture supportive and sharing, and concerned for each other. Such concern of the organisation about the human factors (resources) can help significantly in successful implementation of health; promotion schemes for the workers by supplying adequate oxygen (psychological support and security) to them.

In practice however, programmes for stress management frequently employ a combination of biofeedback, relaxation training, physical aerobic exercise, and cognitive modifications.

Whatever may be the type of the technique employed, without cognitive exercise by oneself, no technique can show positive treatment outcome. Because, in every technique, the individual is helped to learn auto-control. For example, in biofeedback technique, two cognitive mechanisms account for success of treatment (Holroyd, Appel & Andrasik, 1983). These two are changes in self-efficacy, and in locus of control. In biofeedback—when a client feels that his headache could be reduced by controlling muscle tension (locus of control) and that they can do when they develop a belief that they can control their muscles constriction (self-efficacy enhanced) by themselves.

For enhancement of self-efficacy the most popular technique and, recently, most frequently employed technique is called counselling. Counselling can help developing psychological control to monitor effective coping. This is through imparting training to develop self-confidence, self-efficacy, and adequate self-esteem. Also, to train the clients to focus more attention to their own positive life resources, viz., stable home environment, stable economic condition, social status and development of regular life style conductive to face stress, viz., food habit, physical exercise, etc. Lack of self-confidence, self-efficacy and self-esteem does not help to apply confrontative coping style. As opposed to avoidant coping style, which may provide a short-term, temporary escape, confrontative coping requires to execute action by the client himself/herself. The latter enables one to be equipped to deal with long-term threats. In addition to one's own personal resources, certain external resources, viz., a good circle of friends, and associates, congenial interaction with others, required economic status, etc. are usually found to be secondary forces in active coping. Needless to mention that utilisation of external forces also depends upon the personality characteristics of the stress minimisers. Individual counselling can help a employee understand his psychological needs, feelings, motives, drives, and also the defences he/she employs and coping strategies selects for facing stress.

The concept, theoretical background, steps in counselling, and procedures for counselling and certain other issues related to counselling—particularly in context to organisational and clinical stress—will now be discussed in the next chapter.

Chapter 5

INTERVENTION THROUGH COUNSELLING : ITS ORIGIN AND DEVELOPMENT ACROSS CULTURE

Counselling services seem to have developed as an offshoot of guidance programme. Initially, guidance programmes were particularly' vocational and educational in nature. The most notable of these are—the first systematic vocational programme launched by Merrill (1895) in San Francisco (cited by Rao. 1981). Thereupon, vocational bureau was established by Williamson (1965) and Patterson (1973) at the University of Minnesota. While catering to guidance needs, the then scientists strongly felt the necessity to supplement their services through suitable tests and adequate techniques. Such that, they urged upon the development of tools for assessing primary mental functions aptitude, interest, and intelligence of the clients seeking such services. But the concept of clinical counselling was not much in vogue at that time.

As reported by Rao (1981), the term 'counselling' was first used by Jesse B. Davis in 1898 who had taken keen interest in educational career counselling and established centre for the same at Detroit. Lightner Witner (1896) founded the first psychological clinic and thus proclaimed the beginning of counselling movement (Rao, 1981).

During the fist half of the 20th century tremendous progress was made in this area by the founding of free clinic in connection with assessment of mental functions and their development by Miner (1909) at the University of Minnesota (Rao, 1981). To establish counselling as a science and to disseminate its application to society, particularly in clinical orientation, a major breakthrough was achieved through the pioneering write-ups of Carl Rogers, e.g., 'Counselling and Psychotherapy' (1942). A remarkable change in character of such services was evident during the second world war (1939—1945) and post-War period. The counselling programme as a part of the 'Army separation and classification' was introduced (1944) and, thereafter, counselling as a part of rehabilitation programme was initiated. Though controversies prevailed even up to 1960s regarding the future of counselling as a specialised field (Brayfield, 1961, 1963), counselling, in due time, got its referred status (Yamamoto, 1963)) after obtaining recognition by the American Psychological Association (APA, 1956). Thereupon counselling psychology has been recommended by the APA as a special division of psychology (earlier the division was designated as counselling and guidance; Rao, 1981). The American Board of Examiners in professional psychology introduced certification and professional examinations separately for counselling psychologists. Even a separate council on counselling psychology was launched first in 1954 (for detail please see Rao, 1981).

Not only in Europe and America, in India too, counselling in some form or the other was present since long. Calcutta (now Kolkata) has had taken a pioneering role in the application of psychological principles in the treatment of mentally ill patients. It does not require volumes to weigh the contributions of Dr. Girindra Shekar Bose (G.S. Bose) who being a physician by profession, trained himself in psychoanalysis and initiated its application for the treatment of such people. Dr. Bose the first official proponent of psychoanalysis and founder of the Indian Psychoanalytical Society (1922) at 14, Parsibagan Lane, Kolkata 700 009 assigned this method of treatment an international and scientific character. Later some of his followers, viz. T.C. Sinha (who also set up an institute for psychoanalysis, named SAMIKSHANI), Dhirendranath Ganguly and others continued this trend in Kolkata for the treatment of emotionally disturbed individuals. At the National Institute of Mental Health and Neurosciences (NIMHANS), Bangalore, research has been conducted on parapsychology. As the training procedures which an analyst has to undergo and the methods of psychoanalysis for the treatment of the patients are altogether different from the recently used techniques applied for counselling, detailing of psychoanalysis and its treatment methods seem beyond the scope of this chapter. Chapter on psychotherapy would have some relevance to psychoanalysis. Counselling technique was introduced primarily to help people who were emotionally disturbed. Question remains whether it had been applied in formal method in formal setting, or in formal method within an informal setting, or totally an informal method in an informal setting. Whatever it may be, its application has to depend largely on—(i) the purpose of counselling, (ii) expertise of the counsellor, and (iii) socio-economic norms employed in the life of the counselee.

India has inherited a vast wealth of knowledge from Saints and sages about mental health problems and also about methods of its amelioration. Sages and gurus were serving as counsellors and guides. Traditional healing method is known as instant cure. The Epics and Puranas provide guidance for effective ways of living. The Bhagavad Gita is a masterpiece of psychotherapy; the Atharvaveda is considered as ancient guidebook of psychotherapy. The Nyaya system has analysed the emotional aspects of behaviour along with cognitive interpretations of behaviour (Rangaswami, 1996), while the yogic system provide information on ancient methods of developing physical and mental well-being. Western experts, e.g., Wolberg (1977) considered yoga as a combination of supportive and re-educative type of therapy, whilst Begart (1991) considered these as methods of providing insight into one's personal identity. In India, clinicians are of the opinion that these methods are based on the principle of learning and behaviour modification (Balodhi and Mishra, 1983)—thus yogic methods have both preventive and curative implications (Verma, 1995).

In meditation, in its final stage, the individual passages through a trance state through self-suggestions which produces a strong therapeutic effect. The origin of this can be traced back to the individual's aspects of faith (Alexander, 1979; Hoch, 1977). Meditation—though derived from Asian psychological methods (Kabat-Zinn, 1990; Ramdass, 1971)—has become popular all over the world, so much so that it has been accepted as supplementary technique for psychotherapy, called metatherapy by Goleman (1971). In America, meditation is practised more particularly in stress management programmes and in cognitive behavioural therapy (Meichean Baum, 1994).

Psychotherapy in India leans on its spiritual heritage (Dhairyam, 1961). Such leaning on spiritual heritage was reported to be present in the Western psychotherapy as well. Dhairyam (1961), in this context opined that Western psychotheraphy is based on Judaeo-Christian tradition. Likewise, experts in the West, e.g., Lazarus (1981), and those in India, viz., Rangaswami (1961), Mishra (1988), Nathawat and Khan (1995) have long before focussed on the importance of spirituality in psychotherapy and behaviour therapy (Miller and Martin, 1988). The Spirituality has been prevailing in counselling-psychotherapy universally.

Techniques like Progressive Muscular Relaxation, Autogenic Training and Desensitisation developed in the West are similar in principle and practices with Indian systems like *Pranayam*, *Shavasana* and meditation (Paranjee, 1984; Mishra, 1984; Rangaswami, 1996) employed to avoid existential sufferings and maintain tranquility and mental peace.

Over the past few decades counselling has gained overwhelming acceptance from different sectors of our society; still, compared to the strength of population in India (1.23 billion = 123 crores, in 2011), the nature and degree of awareness are relatively low, particularly in the rural sectors of India. Sub-specialities have developed to serve in different settings like schools and colleges, corporate organisations, mental health clinics, community agencies, rural centres and so on. Several theoretical approaches to counselling are in vogue. However, fundamental modifications of theoretical construct of counselling may be needed to suit the culture-originated problems. Cheatham (1990), in this context, first commented on the danger of counselling that is culturally insensitive.

Cultural issues in counselling will now be discussed in Chapter 6.

Chapter 6

CULTURAL ISSUES IN COUNSELLING

Professional counselling is an art based on scientific approaches. The Art and Science of counselling need to be implemented with reference to the client's surrounds, especially when a counsellor is concerned with clinical population.

To facilitate better understanding of human behaviour, psychology has to be anchored in its psychosocial and sociocultural systems. Child rearing practices, for e.g., foster security and trust in the child; thereupon, family system, larger social system (group interaction) and cohesive interdependence assure protection in the individual. Emotions, needs, drives, and motives are relational. Therefore, psychological problems experienced by individuals are mostly disorders of relationship (from relationship generates expectations) with fellow beings. Concern about developmental phases of a given client, during counselling, is to ensure whether child rearing practices fostered insecurity and mistrust in the child, as a result of which the child has been manifesting symptoms later in life. Content of expectations and methods of its fulfilment vary largely from one country to the other. Like many other cultures, Indian culture is also influenced by its social reality and cultural specificity (Dhairyam, 1961; Kakar, 1981). Mishra (1988) stated that the self, states of consciousness, and yoga are the areas in which traditional Indian thoughts contribute to understanding psychological processes of a man. Accordingly, to deal with problem behaviour, culture specific phenomena requires special attention (Misra and Agarwal, 1985). This would provide better insight into the cultural realities, and culturally congruent perspective of behaviour-pathology.

Self has been viewed as a major concept in Indian psychology in understanding behaviour. Accordingly, self-efficacy, self-control, and self-regulation are the main constructs used for having a clear idea about one's self. Rangaswami (1994) had delineated very clearly how the Indian world view differs from that of the West. The Indian world view, such as, *dharma, karma* (sacrifice and sharing), self-esteem, spirituality, and the ultimate goal in life are the most important theoretical constructs in understanding human behaviour. The spiritualistic nature of man is guided by the doctrine of *Dharma*. Dhairyam (1961), thus, has long before advocated that psychotheraphy in India has to lean on spiritual heritage of India. Such a view has also been propounded by Sinha (1984) where he expressed his anguish stating that it is of course unfortunate that many a times psychologists hesitate to talk about our own heritage.

According to the *Karma* theory, the past, the present and the future deeds form a continuum in our lives. The past action (deeds) determine the nature and course of the present behaviour, and the present deeds, in turn, pave way to the future behaviour. This, in other words, focussed on the concept of life after death. The doctrine of *karma* acts as an anchor in human life which, ultimately, provides security in life. If however, an individual develops a feeling that somehow he has deviated from following the doctrine of *karma* through his life activities, such belief in our socio-cultural framework, on the other hand, acts a seed giving rise to feelings of guilt, injustice, insecurity etc. Surrender has been used, by and large, as a coping mechanism; the deterministic concepts decide upon the locus of control. For detail of the non-Western perspective in psychology, the reader is referred to Sinha (1981), and Ghorpade and Kumar (1988).

We are greatly influenced by our family tradition in particular and societal conditions in general. Of course, it does not necessarily mean that persons from a given community will always have common culture and heritage. There may be considerable diversity among people, say, in language, religion, and in many such other attributes even though they all belong to the same culture. Apart from different communities; there are also differences amongst members of the same family in their life style and idiosyncracies.

India is a very big laboratory for experimentation since it is structured with multi-religion and multi-lingual sensibilities. Communication problems make it difficult, and sometimes awkward too, for many clients to explain their problems and to receive adequate help they require. Since effective communication is crucial to the provision of counselling, the counsellor needs be well-versed in the language the counselee uses as medium of communication. Likewise, the counsellor must be acquainted with the religious norms of the counselee, to provide, appropriately, responsive form of solution to his/her problem. Thus, the counsellor is to be provided with cultural sensitivity training so that the counselee can obtain maximum satisfaction and gain from his/her assistance. Cultural gaps often lead to misunderstanding and ill-advised management/treatment strategies (Hughes, 1993).

It is also vital for a counsellor to have awareness of how certain issues like, gender, ethnicity, spirituality, patterns of emotional interaction etc. act as determinants in attributing different meanings (constructs) to life events. For example, in olden-days, gender discrimination used to prevail quite significantly in Indian families where the male child used to be considered superior. Accordingly, males used to be provided with educational, occupational and various other life opportunities, whereas females used to be deprived totally from enjoying such facilities; females didn't have adequate exposure too for social interaction. The situation, now, has changed radically so much so that females are, by and large, getting all such opportunities to establish themselves independently. However, even now in some families such gender discrimination appears to prevail, which, of course, is very unfortunate. Such discrimination has its impact onto emotionality of the females.

Interaction pattern in Indian families and development of emotionality show wide variation compared to those that prevail in the West. As an illustration of how cultural expectations infuse family and group experiences, it may be mentioned that Indian family interaction style encourages more of dependency in decision—making rather than helping a child to be independent, which, in later stages of life, affect adversely his/her life interaction—particularly when he/she requires to take decisions alone. In traditional Indian families, where extended family system prevails, a person's individuality is absorbed into the collective family community. Thus, when a person in afflicted by emotional problems, it is likely to be perceived as a family (mini-community) problem which, consequently, affects the entire family. Individuals have had little or no input into the choice of a marriage partner in traditional Indian culture, where marriages are arranged by parents and other family members. Though the situation is changing now, it is causing lots of problems in life adjustments of both the younger generation as well as that of the seniors. It must not mean, however, that Indian family interaction style has no positive outcome. Actually, it provides a sense of 'We' feeling amongst the members and thus prepares them mentally to share with each other their well and woes. Such an affectionate bondage amongst the members of Indian family is really unique.

Not only regarding single culture phenomenon, a clinician-counsellor has to be aware of possible hazards originating from the sub-cultural, bicultural/multicultural issues in counselling. In Indian e.g., sub-cultural variations are evident in our life-style and also in symptom manifestations (Chattopadhyay and Chattopadhay, 2009); a professional counsellor in clinical set-up has to be well-versed in the counsellee's societal conditions and cultural norms. Many of our clients report life experiences which are admixture of more than one cultural tradition.

Decision-making process is an outcome of one's meaning-making process which evolves through family interaction and cultural influences. Therefore, no single interaction approach/strategy is equally effective across all populations and life situations. Effectiveness of counselling is enhanced when the counsellor uses techniques, strategies and fixes goals which are consistent with the life-style and cultural values of a given client. Cheatham (1990) commented on the danger of counselling/psychotherapy that is culturally insensitive. Culture-specific strategies in counselling have been detailed elsewhere (Sur, 1990).

Many people who live in a different culture than that of their own encounter personal identity problem. For example, dimensions of spiritualism, individualism, emotionality, thoughts, beliefs, etc. are likely to influence people differently, for example, those who are born and brought up in Europe and those who are born and brought up in the Eastern part of the globe but settled in Europe later in life. Deep influence of culture and its effects remain intact even if the person migrates to another culture (Suhail, 2000; Bose, 1997; Bhattacharya. 1986). Hale and Pinninti (1994) reported that Asians living in the UK reported delusions of ghost possession, though such delusions are uncommon in Britain. This is because such delusions are common in South-Asian countries. Of course, shared themes in symptoms may be found in some cases due to similar environmental experiences. Suhail (2000), for example, suggested that the Indians living in the UK and the British group did not differ regarding the types of different hallucinations. In this context, Kirowsky (1985) opined that some indications of cultural inheritance is evident in symptoms after a close scrutiny, even though, apparently, symptoms might appear similar. For example, thought problems leading to delusions, and perceptual problems leading to hallucinations may be relatively universal manifestations in schizophrenia due to underlying organic dysfunction. Even then, mistrust, for example, as a theme in delusions varies in thematic elements according to the group culture. For example, in Suhail's (2000) study, majority of both the British and Indians living in the UK reported delusions of persecution, but Indian patients excelled in the frequency of persecutory delusions. Likewise, greater persecutory ideas were found in actual inhabitants of India, in another study (Kala and Wig, 1982) as well. Rao (1966), long back suggested that, in Indian children, childhood is characterised by repression of hostility; family is involved in developing such themes in delusions as a high premium is placed on Indian children who obey their elders, whereas expression of aggression hardly receives any encouragement. Tateyama *et al*, (1993) reported that themes of direct persecution were more conspicuous amongst German patients than amongst Japanese patients. The latter showed greater themes related to delusions of reference.

However, it is useful to remember that cultural attitudes develop and change over time. Modern technological development, high speed mass media for dissemination of information have resulted in easy intermixture of cultures from different parts of the world. No doubt such broadening of vision has some healthy outcome, but there is always a lurking danger of developing feelings of insecurity, indecisiveness, value conflicts, emotional instability in individuals—particularly in adolescents and young adults on account of losing hold of roots. Also, such rapid technological and social changes further widens the generation gaps between the seniors and the young. Modification in affective-cognitive domain of the individual can be done through scientific techniques of counselling, provided the counsellor is well aware of the cultural roots of the counselee.

Discontentment has been voiced by clinicians not only in India but in other parts of the globe too, regarding the use of certain given techniques of counselling across culture. Therefore, attempts have been made to implement culture-specific strategies. For example, in Canada and in Europe, attempts have been made to incorporate their social life experiences in their therapeutic endeavours. In the Third World perspective, the issues concerning implementation of indigenous culture specific concepts in psychotherapeutic intervention strategies were raised by Sinha and Holtzman (1984). The need for developing Indian psychotherapeutic model has been stressed upon by Sethi (1977) and some directions for indigenisation of psychotherapy have been given by many Indian stalwarts (Surya and Jayaram, 1964; Neki, 1973, 1976, 1979; Sinha, 1983) long before.

Balancing of personality traits *(Gunas)*, viz., *Satavic*, *Rajasic*, and *Tamasic* has been emphasised in Indian epics. Detailing of these is beyond the scope of this book. However, balancing of Indian philosophical concepts of personality with the Indian indigenous psychotherapeutic techniques have been delineated well by Rangaswami (1996). Individual personality characteristics, viz., independence-dependence, responsibility taking-avoidance, interactive-withdrawn etc. are largely determined by cultural forces. In contrast to the West, Indian clients are, by and large, found to be dependent and support-seeking with a tendency to discard ego boundaries (Rangaswami, 1996) and desire the counsellor's direct involvement in decision-making process. Therefore, need for culturally sensitive mode of therapeutic transactions has been urged by many. For example Pande (1968), opined that "Western psychotherapy" is an institution of the Western society. The same view is applicable in context to counselling as well. In Indian set up, therapeutic relationship has been described as '*Guru-Chela*' relationship (Dhairyam, 1961; Carstairs, 1965; Neki, 1973) due to cultural compulsions and necessities.

Shamsundar (1997) stated that Neki, perhaps, viewed such relationship as culturally more suitable only with regard to classical psychoanalytical psychotherapy. It is not really so, because, in any type of psychotherapy across culture there has to develop a relationship which is conducive to continue sessions. But Indian clients, mostly show a tendency to lean on the counsellor/therapist with an expectation that the counsellor/therapist will provide them with ready resolution to their problems. Thus, it becomes an additional responsibility on the part of the counsellor/therapist to see that the client/patients can come out from such cultural ingredients of dependency. Had there been no such dependency, perhaps the nature of problems the clients report would have different connotations altogether. Personality inadequacy out of perceived deprivation in receiving support from parents and such other significant figures often get reflected in the therapeutic/counselling sessions. Manifestation of symptoms—like those of somatoform disorders—is mostly an outcome of such unfulfilled need to depend.

Cultural factors influence the process and outcome of counselling—the most important is resistance. During psychological distress, some clients, mostly Indian clients, are mostly found reluctant to turn up for formal professional sources of assistance. Not only for clinical counselling, for educational, vocational and other similar matters too, they show reluctance to receive professional assistance. This is because many of out clients even today, no matter whether educated, or illiterate, rich or poor, are apprehensive that formal consulation will designate them as mentally ill, which of course, is totally a wrong idea they possess. They prefer to rely on informal assistance easily available from family members, elders in the society, and the head of different religious institutions and so forth. In some cases, though the family members feel the need for formal counselling, the client does not; out of family pressure, they become partially motivated to receive such assistance just on a trial basis and expects some miraculous outcome within one or two sessions, even though the problem is a longstanding one. The counsellor, in such cases, cannot implement and complete a set of techniques, because of the client's irregular attendance. The outcome of such unwholesome programme is mostly unsatisfactory. However, the counsellor can help the client to be motivated within a few initial sessions, provided the counsellor has adequate expertise to break such resistance.

Of course, it must not mean that there is no commonness in counselling strategies across culture. Certain common factors are important regardless of culture. For example, ethical issues and medicolegal aspects. The content of these issues may vary across culture and over time, but that counselling involves ethics and legal issues is universally true. Furthermore, professionals all over the world have tried to find commonness, if any, between concepts used by different experts in therapeutic regime. Mention, thus, may be made to Tamase (1991) who made an unique attempt to combine Eastern and Western frameworks. Tamase did not agree with Erikson's view of labelling of development period as being focussed on a particular task. Erikson has labelled, for example, early childhood (2-4 yrs), as a stage of developing a sense of autonomy. Tamase, on the contrary, opined that different cultures are supposed to focus on different tasks at different stages of development, instead of rigidly being fixed on one particular issue only. For example in Africa, Japan, or in South America the goal of this period is not autonomy (Ivey *et al, 1997)*, but rather a sense of connectedness to the caregiver. Network of relationship with caregivers is most important in finding an individual's unique pathway in life adjustment. However, despite such differences in the use of terminology in designating different developmental stages of life, there is commonness amongst professionals across culture in acknowledging the impact of childhood interaction in developing symptoms later on in life.

Chapter 7

COUNSELLING : CONFUSIONS OVER RELATED NOMENCLATURE

The term counselling, no doubt, has been very popular in the present era. It is being used very widely in modern society. But unfortunately, the term counselling is being loosely used, and the method employed is also mostly unscientific. Consequently counselling, as an intervention strategy, is going to lose its significance to the public. It is true that scientific techniques of counselling, too, contains advice giving components, but for that, mere advice giving is not the essence of counselling. Likewise, misconceptions still prevail, even amongst professionals, regarding the differences between the popular use of the term 'counselling' and casual observation and suggestions giving advice, persuasion, guidance and the like on the one hand, and scientific and professional application of the terms in clinical counselling and psychotherapy on the other. Confusions on nomenclature regarding counselling and its related terms has already been depicted by Rao (1981) long before but the term counselling has been very popular recently and thus has increased its probability of misuse and confusions; to overcome this, it will be better to specify what counselling is not.

Assistance

The connotation of the term 'counselling' implies assistance. But any act of assistance giving is not counselling. Counselling is an assistance giving process following scientific methods imparted by a trained professional expert to a needy individual with a responsibility of helping the individual to attain self-sufficiency.

Advice

The process of communication varies between advice and counselling. In general, advice connotes a sort of conviction that what is to be done is told. In this sense, advice involves imposition. But in counselling there is no scope for imposition. Secondly, in advice giving situations, the adviser is assumed to be superior and the person receiving advice is expected to accept the advice. In counselling such a notion of superiority-inferiority does not exist. Thirdly, advice seeking implies a sense of shrinking responsibility, on the part of the client, in inquiring into the matter on hand; because it is assumed that it is sufficient to follow whatever is advised. But in counselling, the client cannot shrink such responsibility in understanding his/her ownself and in taking decision independently (ultimate aim of counselling). Fourthly, in advice giving there need not necessarily be any readiness on the part of the person receiving advice to understand matters related to the future action. But in counselling, the individual has to analyse and synthesise his feelings and actions and thus has to consider all future consequences to understand himself in totality in relation to his environment. Fifthly, advice giving may not necessarily follow a scientific process. It may be over in a single occasion. But counselling, being more scientific, requires several sessions and even follow up. Thus, counselling is more time taking than advice giving. Sixthly, person receiving advice may not show any change in his behaviour even after seeking advice repeatedly (being dependent), but in counselling the aim is to see that the person who requires counselling becomes independent in problem-solving and thus reduces the frequency of seeking help in solving his/her problems (being independent and mature). Seventhly, in advice the decision has to be taken by the giver, whereas, in counselling, ordinarily, the decision has to be taken by the recipient.

In sum, counselling, in a multidimensional developmental orientation, helps the recipient to become self-sufficient. It enhances his/her emotional, social and cognitive development. In this sense, professionally trained counsellors' services are developmental, therapeutic, and preventive in nature. Scientific counselling aims at a long cherished goal, particularly in clinical set-up.

Direction

It implies a sense of command; it is authoritarian in character and connotes an expectation of obedience. The very idea of authority, command, and obedience are completely alien to the counselling situation. In counselling, on the other hand, the client is counselled for understanding the cause(s) of his problem(s), to use his/her own directions to solve the problem(s), and also to face the consequences.

Instruction

Like direction, instruction too, is usually obligatory (for the advisee) with an expectation on the part of the advisor that, the person to whom the instruction is given will follow it. In counselling, on the other hand, no such obligation works as because the counsellors place the realities to the client with a view to prepare the client to decide upon the future course of action.

Education

Education aims at an all-round development of the individual. It aims at bringing out the best in an individual. As in counselling, the client is helped to obtain a realistic understanding of himself/herself—counselling is a form of specialised eduction, extended in a more scientific manner. But, all education is not counselling. Education aims to develop insight into an individual. How to know that the client has developed insight into his problem? In Indian cultural context, development of insight would mean that the counselee is in a position to control his impulses in satisfying his urges by differentiating between *'Shreyas'* and *'Preyas'* (Dave, 1991). 'Shreyas' means which is good for the individual and also that it is suitable for the individual in terms of his/her cultural norms. *'Prayas'*, on the other hand, means that what the individual wants irrespective of whether it suits him or is good for him. In this regard, a professional counsellor requires a considerable amount of professional skills to help the client developing a sense of objectivity in him, i.e., responsiveness without any personal bias.

Guidance and Counselling

The term 'guidance' is commonly used in relation to 'counselling'. Guidance means to provide assistance to make intelligent choice and proper decision. Guidance essentially consists of giving information. No doubt information is necessarily given in counselling too, but only information giving is not counselling. The most important and popular type of guidance is educational, and vocational guidance.

Both in India and abroad, systematic guidance used to be offered by some philanthropic persons who were motivated to help the needy. As in the USA, Frank Parason (known as Father of Vocational Guidance), so in Mumbai, India, Hosuarg Mehta and Batiliboi have been acclaimed as the first civic leaders of the guidance movement in the Parsi Panchayat Bureau of Bombay (Mumbai) (Dave, 1991). Thereupon H.P. Mehta and Perin Mehta became the first official proponents in giving guidance movement a national (Dave, 1991) and scientific character. Likewise, in India, the guidance movement got is impetus in 1938-1939 when G.S. Bose, the then Head of the Department of Psychology, Calcutta University set-up a section on Applied Psychology in the said department to conduct research in vocational and educational fields using psychological test findings.

Both these terms—guidance and counselling—are mutually related processes, but they are not synonymous. Guidance is a relatively more comprehensive process and counselling is a very specialised function of it. The counselling is the nucleus of overall assistance giving through guidance. In other words, guidance programme, in any form, focusses on, or may be said to culminate, when necessary, in counselling process. Counselling helps the person to weight his cognitive assets and limitations and thus to see a realistic picture of himself. The term counselling in Hindi means *'upbodhan'* (Dave, 1991) , which is derived from the word *'both'*, means knowledge/ enlightment. Thus, counselling connotes the act of imparting all-round enlightment to an individual. Counselling in this sense, is technical in nature.

In sum, compared to guidance, counselling includes diverse areas, has problem-solving orientation and mostly a clinical implication. In this respect one might suggest that counselling is a form of psychotherapy. Let us examine now the similarities and differences, if any, between counselling and psychotherapy.

Counselling and Psychotherapy

Still now there are professionals who think of psychotherapy as psychoanalytic psychotherapy only. But recent use of the term behaviour therapy perhaps creates a difference between psychotherapy—particularly depth psychotherapy—and counselling. One becomes more confused when client-centred approach is referred to as both counselling and psychotherapy. However, there are authors both in support of and against regarding the differences between counselling and psychotherapy. Let us examine some such viewpoints.

The semantic characteristics of these two words are not strictly the same (Rao, 1981). That could be the reason that the person who seeks help through psychotherapeutic intervention is customarily designated as 'patient' than the one who receives services through counselling. The latter is referred to as 'client' That is, patients taken for psychotherapy have deep level, serious emotional problems unlike the clients who come for counselling. In case of the latter, the disturbances are not serious enough to incapacitate, or to interfere development of his/her potentialities. The problems of such clients are mostly conscious, for example, educational counselling, vocational counselling. Psychotherapy, on the other hand, is exclusively concerned with the problems emanating from the deep-lying personality components of the person and are primarily unconscious (Patterson, 1973). Countary to this, some of the professionals are of the opinion that such distinctions cannot be sustained on close scrutiny as because counselling also deals with all the domains of personality—cognitive, connative, and affective, and thus closely approaches psychotherapy. Since affective components are involved, it might require help from an expert who is a professional-clinical counsellor to deal with the unconscious phenomenon of the client. When counselling does not deal with affective domain of the client scientifically, then it might become more of an advice giving, not actually counselling. Mere advice giving is admittedly most differentiated from counselling or psychotherapy either. A trained psychotherapist can render counselling services, if required. For untrained, non-clinical persons (i.e., without any background of psychology at the PG level and post-PG specialisation in clinical psychology) it would be hazardous to take clients/patients for counselling or psychotherapy either, because such services require thorough analyses and syntheses of the deep level affective problems, in terms of, say, defences used, and mode of coping and conflict resolution etc., which can never be dealt with through common-sense advice.

Supportive counselling is required sometimes. Psychiatric treatment, viz., pharmacotherapy is applicable (medicines prescribed by physician, preferably a psychiatrist) for controlling overexcitability, hyperactivity etc. Supportive counselling provides reassurance. In such cases, many a time family members of the client may have to be involved during the intervention session. Discussion, planning, and execution of the intervention strategy along with the psychiatrist/physician may lead to a quick recovery in some cases. Such an arrangement for a joint effort in implementation of therapeutic strategy is relatively less in our country. Since the term counselling has acquired different shades of meaning, to make sure what clinical counselling is, let us examine now some of the other related nomenclature.

Debates on the similarities and differences between counselling and psychotherapy are endless. Divergent views have been reported in the literature which ranges from no difference (e.g., Jacobs, 1996; Strawbridge,. 1999; O'Brian, 1996) to that of very significant differences (Dryden, 1996; Harvie-Clark 1999)—such diametrically opposed views have made controversy unavoidable, and more so when some of the authors have suggested (e.g., Jacobs, 1996) that these two terms are interchangeable. Many of these controversies, of course, help us to go into the core of what actually clinical counselling and psychotherapy are. Let us see now the similarities and differences, if any, between clinical counselling and phychotherapy :

DIFFERENCES	**SIMILARITIES**
Depth of the Problem and Duration of Intervention	
(1) Clinicial counselling has been restricted to problems which are situational, specific and conscious, i.e., reality oriented, whilst psychotherapy is concened with problems which are interpersonal, embedded and unconscious, and is thus much more brain storming. The counsellors are concerned with relief of immediate discom-	(1) No clear distinctions exist between clinical counselling and psychotherapy (Jacobs, 1996).

Contd.

fort, while psychotherapists are concerned with total life experience of the patient (Einzig, 1989).	
Issues about Power and Status	
(2) Higher status of practices is termed psychotherapy, and relatively lower status counselling (Dryden, 1996).	(2) From the point of view of practice no such useful distinction can be made (O'Brian, 1996).
Techniques Employed	
(3) Distinction is made between psycho-dynamic counselling and psychoanalytic psychotherapy (Harvie-Clark, 1999) and behaviour therapy, cognitive therapy and so on.	(3) Client-centred therapist and cognitive therapist—these two terms may be interchangeably used, but finally it leads to confusion (Naylor-Smith, 1994).
Nature of Profession	
(4) Psychotherapy has been sometimes associated with medical profession, and counselling with non-medical profession (Dryden, 1996).	(4) Such differences have been denied altogether by Rogers (1961) and later by others, e.g., Lewis, 1970.
Expertise	
(5) A counsellor cannot be a psychotherapist but a psychotherapist can be a counsellor (Nayak, 1997) as psychotherapist is a specially qualified expert. Clinical psychologists must have a basic PG degree in psychology, and M. Phil or equivalent in clinical psychology. They undergo a 2-year fulltime internship course in psychodiagnostic, psychopathology, psychophysiology, neuropsychology, in addition to theoretical curriculum, to render counselling or psychotherapeutic services. Without any PG degree in psychology and clinical training (also psychoanalyst has a rigorous training including self analysis) one is not competent to render clinical counselling or psychotherapeutic services either.	(5) For a non-clinical setup, counsellors who have received training for educational and/or vocational counselling and the like may be able to render services in the related areas; such training must also be, necessarily, recognised with adequate accreditation. But such professionals are not competent to provide intervention which requires depth interpretation, for example, marital counselling. However, trained psychotherapist is competent enough to cover all the above mentioned services.

Contd.

<table>
<tr><th colspan="2">Accreditation</th></tr>
<tr><td>(6) Differences are evident in providing accreditation to the professionals. Relevant, specialised and recognised body should provide such accreditation keeping at par with the nature of the training received by the professionals. For example, British Psychological Society enrols for Counselling and U.K. Council for Psychotherapy. In India Girindra Sekhar Clinic, Kolkata (affiliated to American Psychoanalytical Society) enrols for psychoanalysis only. Similarly, Indian Association of Clinical Psychologists (IACP) recognises clinical psychologists only.</td><td>(6) Some of the organisations/institutions, viz., Rehabilitation Council of India provides accreditation to non-clinical professionals and clinical psychologists.</td></tr>
<tr><th colspan="2">Transference and Counter Transference</th></tr>
<tr><td>(7) When greater dependency and/or regression are evident, 'the work may be viewed clearly as psychotherapy' (Naylor-Smith, 1994).</td><td>(7) In any such remedial transaction, transference has to take place. To deal with the problems of transference and counter tansference, expertise of the consultant is equally essential, no matter whether he/she is a counsellor or a psychotherapist.</td></tr>
<tr><th colspan="2">Frequency of Session and Nature of Interpretation of Symptoms</th></tr>
<tr><td>(8) With more frequent sessions, more focus on the dream analyses, and analyses of phantasies—the intervention strategies turnout to be psychotherapeutic (Naylor-Smith, 1994).</td><td>(8) It implies that, (from the Naylor-Smith's, 1994 view) less frequent Sessions and no focus on unconscious matter—make the intervention strategy counselling.</td></tr>
<tr><th colspan="2">Who Receive Services</th></tr>
<tr><td>(9) When a patient is given services, it is called psychotherapy, when non-clinical population is rendered such services it is usually called counselling.</td><td>(9) This is not necessarily true always. For example, client-centred therapy of Rogers (1961). It is called therapy and the person receiving help/intervention is called client. Also, client centred (person-centred) approach is referred to as both counselling and psychotherapy.</td></tr>
</table>

Contd.

Stigma	
(10) Psychotherapy focusses attention almost exclusively upon pathology and medical treatment (Williamson, 1950) and thus gives an impression to the public that receiving psychotherapy would mean that the person is mentally ill. Thus, they show strong resistance to receive such services. Many people actually receive psychotherapy, but publicly uses the term counselling to be stigma-free. Counselling in prima-facie envisages a non-medical orientation and thus the term has been popular and more easily acceptable to the public. Unless such orientation can be changed, etymological meaning does not really make any difference.	(10) In India, particularly in some segments of population, there prevails an idea that any intervention is medically oriented (prescription bound). They expect a drug prescription from even a psychotherapist/counsellor. In this sense, counselling or psychotherapy does not make any difference to them. Likewise, taking any drug, e.g., a night sedation, does not exclude a person to be a subject for psychotherapy or counselling.
Training Imparted	
(11) Psychotherapists require rigorous training, though self-analysis is not mandatory for all. Though, in counselling, personnel training has been mandatory only recently, the whole process of counselling is less rigorous, less time consuming.	(11) Some authors do not agree to such significant differences (Palmer, 2000).
Intricacies of the Methods Employed and Aim of Treatment	
(12) Considering the aim of treatment and intricacies of the methods employed, trained psychotherapist believe in significant differences in the methods employed— (i) psychotherapy aims at restructuring of personality in a radical way (Rao, 1981) whereas counselling is more reeducative in nature. The latter is done in a much less robust way; (ii) since psychotherapy aims restructuring of personality, it is seriously concerned with the patients' psychopathology. Thus restructuring of personality requires a de-	(12) Lewis (1970), however, denied altogether any such differences, which could be made based on the training of the expert. Until Rogers, though there prevailed a belief that psychotherapist should have a medical background, Rogers (1962) exploded these myths. Thus, psychotherapists and counsellors need not have medical training. *Contd.*

tailed account of childhood events and experiences with a view to trace the origin/roots of the problems the patients complaint of. Counselling, on the other hand, aims to solve immediate problems of the client; so it is less probing in nature, more of a supportive type to help the client restore his/her decision making process and self-understanding. It is not concerned about pşychopathology, particularly when it is not medically oriented, e.g., educational counselling, career counselling, vocational counselling, etc.	
Set-up	
(13) A clinical set-up is indispensable for psychotherapy, whereas it is not necessary for counselling.	(13) The major objective of all counselling in clinical set-up like that of psychotherapy is to help the client achieve healthy development, optimum adjustment and maximum happiness. The individual becomes self-dependent, self-directed—with a feeling of self-sufficiency (Dave, 1991).
Time	
(14) Psychotherapy demands a long term commitment unlike counselling.	(14) When counselling is clinical in nature, it is as time-consuming as psychotherapy. If there is any difference in time involvement that is more due to the method employed. For example, short term psychotherapy and/or brief counselling. Otherwise for depth interpretation, both require long time commitment. Again, behaviour therapy as a type of psychotherapy is less time taking. Of course, behaviour therapy is different in nature compared to depth psychotherapy. The present issue under discussion is not to compare, with respect of time, between different types of psychotherapy, but to compare methodological issues pertaining to counselling and psychotherapy.

Code of Ethics

(15) Both the counsellor and the psychotherapist must belong to a registered professional learned body which has a set of published code of ethics.

In sum, depending upon the purpose, the setting where it is applied, and the methodology employed, one might designate a particular intervention, either as counselling or as psychotherapy. If applied in a non-clinical setting with an aim to solve immediate query which does not require inquiry about probable pahology that might be involved (just with an end to provide a guideline for immediate future), then, it may be designated as counselling; namely, career counselling, educational counselling, vocational counselling, etc. It has a broader perspective but narrower vision. On the other hand, when intervention is applied in a clinical set-up with the aim to probe into the psychopathology behind the manifested symptoms, to provide insight into the problem(s), with the aim of restructuring personality for long-term future, then it may be labelled as psychotherapy. It has a narrower perspective, pinpointed/specific aim but much wider vision. However, type of psychotherapy applied, for example, supportive psychotherapy, psychoanalytically oriented psychotherapy and so on vary depending upon the psychological status of the patient.

Chapter 8

COUNSELLING : THEORETICAL FRAME OF REFERENCE

Different theories of counselling have been advocated by different theoreticians and clinicians. These are based on varying concepts of human personality development, its structure and dynamics. No single theory, perhaps, has so far been able to encompass all the aspects of counselling. However, some of the representative approaches, relevant to the present context, will now be depicted briefly.

Psychodynamic

This approach focusses on uncovering of unaware impulses and motivating forces that drive one towards action. Such unveiling aims to (a) discover an association between the past and the present, (b) develop insight into the problems client/patient reports. However, wide variations are noted amongst scholars and clinicians in designating such association. To mention a few, sexual development, particularly oedipal complex for example, has been often focussed by orthodox psychoanalysts, whereas supporters of attachment theory (Bowlby, 1988), and object relations orientations (Winnicott, 1988), concentrate on matters related to the infancy and childhood. Supporters of the rational-emotive therapy hold that the very attempt to make past as determining factor for the present is irrational (Davis, Eschalman, and McKay, 1995). Again, clinicians with feminist orientation (e.g., Okun, 1992) focus on cultural gender role influences onto our life activities, whilst Jungians attribute cultural 'archetype' as determinant of our present behaviour. Despite such divergent views, a convergence in opinion regarding the central importance of unconscious is found to prevail amongst many of the advocates of this approach. Nevertheless, the concept of unconscious has been severely criticised by many stalwarts. Some clinicians are of the opinion that psychodynamic theory needs to be contrasted with psychoanalytic theory. The latter refers specifically to Freudian orientation, whereas the former has a broader perspective. Nevertheless, some of the supporters of the latter approach consider that psychoanalytic theory has laid the foundation for advancement of many of the counselling techniques developed latter.

The classical psychoanalytic techniques consist of bringing repressed desires, wishes, and complexes to the conscious level. Dream material is analysed and used in the explanation of complexes. In the process of analysis the analyst has to successfully deal with the phenomena of resistance and transference. Though psychoanalysis is found to have varying degrees of success with different types of clients, it requires more time—unlike counselling. Furthermore, psychoanalysis has been criticised as the constructs used during the process have not been empirically demonstrable or verifiable. However, the most significant contribution of Freud in this regard cannot be underestimated.

Insight therapies may be reeducative or reconstructive in nature. In the former it is directed toward producing more harmonious self structure. Roger's person-centred approach is an example of insight therapy with re-educative goal (Tucker, 1970). Reconstructive approach helps in gaining insight into the individual's unconscious conflicts which aims at bringing extensive alteration in the individual's character structure (Freudian and other psychoanalytic approaches). Both these approaches differ from the supportive approach which believes in restoring the individual's adaptive capacities by teaching him new ways to maintain control, without probing into the roots of the problem.

For brevity of space, discussion of specifics in favour and against the controversies mentioned above would not be possible. What needs special mention here, however, is that, cultural variability is evident in considering appropriateness of the client's insight into his or her problem.

Developing insight through counselling requires some degree of academic achievement and intellectual efficiency on the part of the client. Otherwise clients may not be in a position to appreciate the counsellor's attempt to help them develop insight into their problems. Some techniques have been found suitable for the uneducated rural population (Hoch, 1963, 1977; Alexander, 1979). Hoch opined that suggestions and spiritual aspect are suitable for the cure of this population. Alexander advocates that faith healing process operates through suggestion. Thus faith provides instant cure. Sometimes, in Indian society, clients fail to make themselves mentally ready to disclose their personal matters essential for developing insight. Moreover, counsellor's attempt to probe into those personal issues of the clients is, many a times, misinterpreted by the client and/or their relatives. This is because they fail to understand the role of the unconscious in their problems; and intricacies of methods employed to reveal the same. Situation may be different with regard to the clients of the Western world. Ivey *et al*, (1997), in this context mentioned that self-disclosure and openness regarding interpersonal matters during therapy is sometimes seen as an expression of immaturity by the clients in the Asian culture. Such misconceptions in some of the clients, however, should in no way undermine the importance of insightful therapy/counselling in clinical set-up. After all, it is the task of the clinician to decide upon which he/she thinks suitable for insightful therapy/counselling and who not. Even now, some of the women in India, in spite of having higher education and financial independence, prefer to be dependent on other members of the family in their daily life interaction. This is because they adhere strictly to the traditional Indian cultural norm, i.e., male domination in social interaction. They are the believers that women must not disclose their discomforts publicly. Such women are found to cooperate more in joint session with their husband/family members, rather than in single session for intervention in analytical orientation. If however, they themselves realise their inadequacy in certain role playing intervention in single session arrangement may not be difficult. Thus, insight becomes a valuable tool leading to new actions and future behaviour.

The client's history of interpersonal relationships and how it gets transferred from the past to the present behaviour are invaluable information to all counsellors. That's how object relations theory develops as an offshoot of psychoanalytic theory. However, theorists (e.g., Bowlby) differ amongst themselves (e.g., Freud, Erikson, Klen and so on) in their view of object relations. For example, Bowlby's ethnological position contrasts markedly with that of Freud's biological determination. What is important for a counsellor to remember is that the structure and functions of families vary widely amongst cultures. In India when joint family system was very much in vogue, care givers for the children used to be their mothers and grandmothers and all others. But the traditional joint family system is weaning, and due to changes in sociocultural outlook, now-a-days many mothers are going out for work and, as such, care givers for the children in nuclear family is mostly an outsider. All such care givers can and do affect children's growth and development differently.

In sum : Psychodynamic components of an individual is a reflection of his/her interaction with family and culture. As an illustration it may be stated that in India we often come across dependent clients though they are grown up by age. In a culture like the USA here autonomy is focussed, excessive dependency has to be dealt with in a different way during counselling than the dependency manifested by Indian clients, in the case of the latter, it might have been encouraged by care givers in some of the families. Dependent client desires to treat the counsellor in a way he has been taught in his family by his/her seniors. But the counsellor cannot encourage such dependency. Such attitudinal differences between the client and the counsellor initially causes lot of problems in counselling sessions and, ultimately, it becomes a hard task for the counsellor to change the attitude of the client to make him independent and self-supported in life.

Psychodynamic approach is not beyond criticisms. It has long been criticised as self-referential and tautologous and irrelevant to many other than middle class clients with high vocabulary (Ivey *et al*, 1997). However, each theoretical framework gives a new perspective, and psychodynamic approach is no exception to it.

Cognitive-Behavioural

Traditionally behavioural and cognitive methods of counselling/therapy though have been applied separately, during the past few decades, theoreticians have found a kinship between these two methods and thus cognitive-behavioural approach has been the treatment of choice for a wide array of clinical problems. In the classical Skinnarian view, direct observable behaviour has been focussed and thus internal speech (cognitions) have not been given adequate attention. Bandura's work may be considered as a turning point in the shift towards a more cognitive orientation. An early statement of the cognitive-behavioural frame work was presented by Cheek (1976) and Meichenbaum (1991). It has brought forward the major changes in establishing such kinship. Later contributions made, in this regard, by Ellis, Beck, Lazarus and others are important in addressing this issue.

Task of a therapist : To define the problem. To fix up goals. To find alternative means to reach the goal. To weigh the costs and effectiveness of each alternative. To decide upon the technique to be executed. To apply the techniques. To ensure that behavioural change is maintained in reality and then follow-up to ensure relapse prevention.

Critics are of the opinion that behaviourism is antithetical to the psychodynamic approaches. Cognitive-behaviour therapy (CBT) in its use of the term cognitive gives primacy to thinking over feeling. How a person develops, in a given culture, particularly regarding the issues of gender is given relatively little attention in CBT theory (Ivey *et al*, 1997). Despite its many positive qualities CBT be used with caution (Kantrowitz and Ballok, 1992).

Let us examine now how CBT can be culturally relevant. We are to control and shape behaviour to suit our cultural and family norms. In doing so, our main task is to choose what behaviour to reinforce, and how and who to decide upon that. It is a collaborative task between the client and the therapist to help the clients appreciate the situation which has been created in a given cultural context. Also, there is a need to realise that we require, sometimes, a shift from individual orientation to that of social context orientation (may be involvement of family members and others required) particularly for deciding upon reinforcing agent(s), and its application in real life situation. Take, for example, training of assertiveness. Assertive behaviour varies between cultures. In Indian culture mostly assertiveness is likely to be misinterpreted by the society as aggressiveness. In actuality assertion must not be equated with aggression. In practice, however, we need to consider the social condition in which our clients live or have lived. Let us consider the difficulties, at times, faced by the counsellors or therapist in Indian context, while imparting assertiveness-training to a meek child. The counsellor/therapist needs to consider a 3-faceted problems that the child may have to deal with, as a consequence of the transition from his behaviour pattern so far to the newly acquired pattern. The 3-faceted problems being : (1) passive (non-violent), non-confrontational stance of such children are reinforced by their family members as opposed to assertive training, creating confusion as to which one is more desirable; (2) in classroom situation, sudden change to assertiveness may be misinterpreated for domination/aggression; (3) this change may be discouraged by some segments of the larger society. Likewise, in those Indian families where gender discrimination prevails, to help a girl to be assertive is normally considered as challenging standard social norms. Assertive training should not be used to teach women a man's style (Kamtrowitz and Ballon, 1992). Cheek (1976) has mentioned several times that cognitive behavioural techniques be applied keeping in mind the gender and culture of the client. Challenging beliefs and thoughts may not fit well with many culture and gender socialisation processes. Kamtrowitz and Ballon (1992) long back reported that Asians have been taught to avoid conflict so as to maintain emotional harmony. "......Women's perceptions have been minimized and misunderstood" (p. 81). Though situation has changed by now, still wide variations are evident in different parts of India and Asia with regard to initiating a shift in cultural norms from that of the past. These issues are to be considered as part of the counselling process. If the counsellor believes in client-centred approach, in such cases, as mentioned above, it creates a dilemma in the counsellor whether he/she has been given complete responsibility to modify the way he/she intends to help the clients to help themselves. Mostly, in India culture, people tend to cope with stressors passively. They try to endure stressor rather than coping with them. In such a scenario, for one, the counsellor's attempt to help the client to cope with the situation may be subject to misinterpretation as being inconsistent with the existing sociocultural norm; and two the client's modified behaviour appears non-adherent to social expectation, the repercussion of which, in turn, could aggravate stress related problems in the client. Such cultural specifications in determining adaptive coping mechanisms should be considered while imparting behavioural-cognitive training through counselling.

With respect to American culture Check (1976) warned that "... assertive training should be oriented to the African-American culture and not make Blacks into White". To take from Check's opinion, for the Indian culture and its rapid occidentalisation, it may be said that care should be taken so that assertive training should not result in the client turning 'Western' as his oriental values may be in conflict with the occidental ones, creating distress in the client. In addition, it is also important to keep in mind that the client should not rigidly stick to his 'Eastern value system' in this fast trend of Westernization, as he will then be a misfit which again will lead to adjustment difficulties. An ideal situation would be a conglomeration of the two worlds where the client is free to hold on to his cultural value system and adopting the more effective aspects of the Western world leading to his/her better adjustment. Likewise, while teaching muscular relaxation training—particularly to the persons of the opposite sex—counsellors in Indian culture must be aware of the boundaries in demonstrating the same to the clients. Many a times, with opposite sex counsellors, our clients show resistance to undergo such demonstration of muscle relaxation alone; they prefer some of their relatives to be present at the time of demonstration. Counsellor has to keep in mind such individual-cultural issues so that stress management programme does not turn out to be a trauma induced session.

Graduated exposure has been found to be highly useful strategy for the treatment of agoraphobia. This is similar to desensitisation except that clients are actually taken into the field for graduated practice. Again, in Indian culture, due to the inhibitions, and stigma related to mental health problems, clients express their unwillingness to take part in such treatment procedures. Thus, multidimensional treatment plan may be useful for multicultural settings. What is most essential here, for a positive outcome, is development of such an attitude in the counsellor which helps him/her to share the sentiment of the client without violating the therapeutic boundaries.

Rational-Emotive Behaviour Therapy (REBT)

REBT originated in 1950s when Albert Ellis, an extremely successful practitioner of psychoanalysis, became dissatisfied with the results he was obtaining on his patients. He later decided to challenge the client's dysfunctional scheme, revealed during therapy and also prescribed behavioural activities to the patients during follow-up (Ellis, 1983). Thus, he punched rational (cognitive) with behavioural theory. In 1994 Ellis changed the name of the age-old therapeutic method from rational-emotive therapy (RET) to rational-emotive behaviour therapy (REBT), because he was of the opinion that application of *in vivo* desensitisation is more of behavioural rather than cognitive, and hence the name REBT. Beck (1997) too, though mostly identified with cognitive methods, used behavioural techniques as well. Thus, it is up to the therapist to decide upon the issue of integration of similar powerful methods in counselling/therapy sessions.

The thrust of REBT is that a man can make himself victim of his own emotions by his own irrational, distorted patterns of thinking. So, REBT focusses more on dysfunctional thoughts of the clients.

Question arises whether REBT is free from cultural influence. Majority of the research workers suggest that REBT does have multicultural relevance. But it all depends upon how efficiently the counsellor conducts the interview. For example,

Scorzelli and Reineke-Scorzelli (1994) found that in Indian population cognitive approach conflicted with the clients' spiritual beliefs, and also with their family and cultural traditions. Even religious beliefs turned out to be a more important factor, and there REBT was less effective. In contrast, REBT was found to be useful for traditional Chinese clients (Chen, 1995). This is because Chinese philosophy values rationality. They emphasise the importance of perception of real events (Chen, 1995). Chen (1995) stressed upon the fundamental issue of building up of therapeutic relationship—here client can develop trust onto the counsellor. Otherwise cognitive approach may turn out to be unsuccessful. In this context Chen (1995) suggested that in REBT, a deep level confrontational style is present. Such confrontational style may not be well accepted by many clients. For example, such confrontational style may be personally and culturally treated as offensive by Chinese clients (Chen, 1995).

In sum, this suggests that the methods of REBT may require modification depending upon the clients' spiritual and cultural orientations.

Counselling, in essence, provides education. *Education*, in Latin, actually means to be aware of from within and to move forward, where *'e'* means from within, and *'duco'* means to go ahead. Thought the meaning of the term education is universal, the contention of life, for which individual is supposed to move varies across culture. Thus, e.g., the contention of the West that the aim of life is to be happy, may be true for us as well, but the means through which individuals will move to reach the goal varies, where Western means may not be validated by Eastern experiences (Basu, 1994). Psychology of individual development is interwined with the psychology of the social development (Sri Aurobindo).

To elevate sufferings, the cognition of the client is most important. For many clients illness behaviour can be managed with spiritual beliefs of the clients; thus effective coping can be implemented. Indian epics, e.g., Puranas, and other literature have provided us guiding principles for counselling in this perspective. For example, the Rig Veda has used the role of offerings and prayer with a view to get relief from sufferings. The Atharva Veda has depicted well about the *Daivya Chikitsa* (heavenly treatment). As mentioned earlier, Indian philosophy emphasises *Karma* doctrine, where surrender as a teachnique has been used to get relief from sufferings. This brings out the importance of spiritual dimension in bringing positive changes in our well-being. Both in the East (e.g., Rangaswami, 1994; Nathwat and Khan, 1995), and in the West (e.g., Rogers, 1984; Young and Marks, 1978) several authors have recognised the influence of religion and its impact on individuals' life style. In context to behaviour therapy, Miller and Martin (1988) have depicted how spiritual perspective can be incorporated in modern psychotherapy for the willing patients.

The Bhagwat Gita, which is an integral part of the Indian epic Mahabharata, has depicted a profile of ideal personality, providing knowledge about the true self. For a comprehensive review on spirituality and psychotherapy in Indian scenario, the interested reader is referred to Rangaswami (1996) and Das (1989).

Case illustration : Male, 26, Graduate in Technology, only son of the family (has 1 married sister), unmarried, employed, came for counselling with the complaints of lack of concentration, low mood, sudden bouts of anger but unable to express it to the appropriate person (occasional outbursts onto his mother, even without any fault of her, followed with repentence by the client), submissive, has difficulty in interacting with strangers, particularly while introducing himself. In-depth interview revealed severe conflict so much so that he felt the need for self-punishment. Whenever he gets an opportunity for life achievement, fails to take initiative to achieve (in spite of having requisite qualities and academic qualifications). On the contrary feels that he should be deprived of such opportunity and be humiliated by others later, because of sinful acts he has done in his life. This, to him, represents a sort of purification (*'Shudhhikaran'* the patient said) of the patient for his misdeeds. Enquiry revealed that he hails from a religious family where his parents meticulously perform religious activities regularly. The contents of his conflicts are—(i) since he believes in religion, he must not have got involved into masturbation, homosexual activities, and voyeurism etc. (ii) Thought he does not deny altogether the need to get married, he is found to be indecisive whenever parents try to arrange for the same. No interaction with girls on his own initiative so far reported. (iii) He believes in Marxism. There too, he faces a conflict as to how his religious belief and faith in God can go hand in hand with his pursuing Marxism. (iv) As a supporter of Marxism, while going out of home, e.g., while going to office, when he worships (*Pranama*) idols, feels that he is neither a devotee of God, nor a believer of Marx truly. Such incongruity in thoughts cause lots of distress in the client psychologically, which he could not reveal to anybody else before.

It is obviously a difficult task on the part of the counsellor to help the client resolve his dilemma, particularly considering the Indian secnario of childhood up bringing and social interaction style of life.

The Existential-Humanistic

The roots of the frame of reference lie in philosophy, the basic of which is to take responsibility for choice and actions in the environment. Existential thought was brought to the awareness of counsellors by May (1969) in the United States. It focusses on the nature and meaning of the client-counsellor relationship. Rogers person-centred counselling approach, particularly the concept of empathy, has popularise this view. The client as human being can determine his own destiny; locus of control and the decision lies within himself. In Rogarian approach, past has not been given importance. But in the humanistic aspect of it, people and their relationship to one another (i.e., environmental determinants) has been focussed. Thus, it is a combination of value and dignity of the clients and also their ability to maintain interpersonal relationship. But question arises—while considering clients' ability to choose and act, can they deny altogether the impact of past?

The most fundamental concept of existentialism is that we are in the world and are constantly interactive with the world. In this interaction others be seen as people rather than objects. Our inability to choose and act to maintain relationship (separateness) results in alienation. The task of a counsellor thus is to enable an alienated client to choose and act in maintaining interaction. Failure to decide upon one's action cause alienation which, ultimately, results in anxiety.

Choice and decision-making process itself can cause a vicious circle. It is known that by choosing one we are denying other possibilities/alternatives. A given client may be in a dilemma whether to choose. Because the client might think that when he chooses, the choice may be incorrect. Such indecisiveness causes anxiety in him. On the contrary, if we refrain from choosing, that too is painful. It is the task of the counsellor to help the client learn that, and to alleviate anxiety, even though, initially, making a choice may be painful, but it is likely to be less painful (anxiety) than the anxiety created by refraining from choosing. Of course, if depends upon the counsellor as to whether he believes that refraining causes more anxiety, or the other way round. This is mentioned because even amongsts existentialists some become pessimistic facing such vicious circle (e.g., Sartre, 1989), whereas humanistic-existentialists take it as an opportunity (e.g., Buber, 1970; Tillich, 1971), for growth. Therefore, the distinction between existential and existential-humanistic approach is based on faith which may sound philosophical to some. The possibilities in the world are perceived as problems (existentialism) or an infinite opportunity (existential-humanistic). As opposed to that of traditional phychodynamic view, where man is perceived as unknowing pledge to the unconscious forces and environmental contingencies, the existential-humanistic approach stressed by Rogers believe that man can decide upon his action and can execute his life plans himself. The task of the counsellor, accordingly, is to assist the client in attaining such intention (self-actualisation) which is natural for every individual.

Rogers' view has been severely criticised. He has not given adequate attention to "reality", Lerner (1992) stated. Also, as Lerner stated, it sounds impractical to ignore totally the influence of "external forces" in forming constructs of reality, which, perhaps, no one can do. Rogers' approach is not free from limitations when applied to multicultural counselling setup (Ivey *et al*, 1997). Furthermore children, adolescents, and less communicable clients cannot be subjected to Rogerian approach as because to understand Rogers' interview, the client requires very high level of cognitive skills. For the clients who require immediate problem solving and also for those who are educationally and economically backward; behavioural, family methods, community methods, and direct approach methods should be the treatment of choice. Though Rogers is acclaimed to be the initiator of the 'client-centred' movement, it is evident that some of the ideas were implicit in the Adlerian approach too. However, Rogers' interviewing skills and humanistic approach have been adopted by many, even by those who believe in eclectic or metatheoretical approach. This is because helping relationship is fundamental here. Of course one might ask that which therapeutic relationship is not helping relationship? Rogers' view is unique in the sense that the counsellor seeks to bring about a better appreciation and a clearer expression of the client's latent inner resources improving upon the client's self-understanding and accelerating his maturity. This helping relationship is essentially an attitude which generates a feeling of acceptance in the client. This attitude does not make a counsellor feel superior to the one who receives help. Also, it implies that the counsellor does not impose his values upon the client. The client realises democratic value of his life.

The existential-humanistic frame of reference have many systems, two of which are (i) Logo Therapy (Frankl, 1985), and Gestalt Therapy (Perls, 1969). But variations are noted, as, for example, Perls took a very different direction from Rogers and Frankl, though later Frankl provides a balancing view between Rogers and that of Perls. Gestalt therapy is centrally concerned with the totaliy of the individual and his existence in the world. It aims to integrate an individual's split-off parts into a complete whole (unique individual). Formation of such a whole also implies inclusion of family and community. It, like Rogers' view, also focusses upon the here-and-now phenomenon. Anxiety, according to Perls (1969), originates when an individual becomes preoccupied with the unknown future ignoring the sure basis of the present (now).

Logotherapy holds that man should not be concerned with what happens but how a phenomenon occurred (individual perception). That is, what is the meaning man attributes to the event which occurs. In this sense then logotherapy is akin to that of cognitive therapy. In fact, Frankl was a forerunner of cognitive-behavioural movement (Mahoney and Freeman, 1985). Thus, this frame of reference provides a bridge between cognitive-behavioural therapies and existential-humanistic approach. Logotherapy seeks to reconcile us to God and Nature, which thus invites lot of controversies. However, for detailed discussion on this issue, the interested reader is referred to Frankl (1959).

Certain limitations of existential-humanistic approach are—though by introducing the concept of spirituality it has got approval from multicultural orientation point of view, its methodology and application technique seem to be slow in solving immediate problems. Thus it may be inappropriate for multicultural clients (Ivey *et al*, 1997). Secondly, this frame of reference totally ignores person-environment transactions in daily life experience which is subject to criticisms for very many reasons. Thirdly, intense preoccupation with individual is a lopsided view of human existence. Fourthly, on the one hand Rogers' view is concerned about the individual only (even ignoring the environmental interaction), whereas the Gestalt therapy approach under the rubric of existential-humanistic frame of reference includes family and culture to assist the client to become a complete and unique whole. This appears in advariance with each other. Nevertheless, family and cultural issues are much involved in the individual, be he a client or a counsellor. Ahia (1991), and deEsche (1991), in this regard stated that individual counselling that fails to include family issues and cultural background is incomplete counselling. However, the mention worthy contribution of existential-humanistic tradition is its strong faith that mankind can perceive infinite possibilities as opportunities in life for his personal growth. Needless to mention that, though this approach sounds easy, like any other counselling method, this also must not be applied by untrained counsellors to save the client from hazardous consequences.

Summing Up

There has been a dramatic change over the last few decades in the field of counselling due to the advent of several new theories and techniques. Counselling/psychotherapy though was initiated with Freudian approach, most of the supporters of Freud later departed from his orientation and introduced new theoretical frame of references. Almost every year so many techniques of counselling are being published in books/journals, that it is confusing, and more so for the learners—as to where to start and where to end. A detailed account of all these appea ˙ eyond the scope of this book. To mention, however, a few of these are—Freud's (psychodynamic approach) contribution; if one thinks of it as the initial force, then subsequently cognitive therapy, behaviour therapy, cognitive-behavioural approach, and existential-humanistic approach, etc. are in force. Of late multicultural counselling has been recognised. Though it recognises and adapts all approaches to counselling, its central focus is on the issue of culture. That is, all problems stem from a cultural base, and thus its alleviation procedure must be culturally oriented. We still need to have more and more awareness and sensitivity to multicultural issues.

Briefly, in a short period of time, theoretical orientation has begun to reshape the field.

In spite of having such a shift of interest in the theoretical frame of reference from the past, no clinician-counsellor perhaps would deny the significant contributions of traditional theories. However, in recent times, the key concern has been circulating around how to integrate these different theoretical frame of references meaningfully. A moot question to a clinician is—for which type of problem of a given client which technique would be suitable, and under what circumstances? Selection of a technique of counselling for a given client requires clinical accumen on the part of the counsellor. One has to develop such accumen through practice of the skills under authentic supervision. Mastering of different basic theoretical issues help in understanding and thereby forming personal style and approach in counselling. Contradictions in basic theoretical issues must be analysed and understood skilfully to form an integrated whole. Such an integration may sometimes be necessary to answer the moot question just raised above that whether one can find any best theory out of all the theories (depicted above), and apply it for a given client under a given circumstance, or one requires to depend upon one theoretical approach only and its methodology.

Eclecticism is still been criticised as it lacks a central theoretical rationale for a counselling procedure. However, such an approach may be useful for some clients. Multimodal counselling of Lazarus (1981) is a form of eclecticism in a more organised way, though it has a bent to behavioural frame of reference. Likewise, Meichenbaum's (1991) cognitive-behavioural approach is another attempt to integrate in a coherent fashion diverse theoretical viewpoints. Again, meditation was not in much use therapeutically, during those days; but now stress management programmes and cognitive-behavioural psychology have adopted meditation as an important method (Davis, Robbins, and McKay, 1995b; Meichenbaum, 1994). Such integration provides a broader scope than traditional approach in counselling.

To conclude, integrated approach is essential to keep pace with the problems our clients mostly report and to help them to ameliorate it; an issue which will be depicted later in this treatise.

Chapter 9

USE OF PSYCHOLOGICAL TEST IN COUNSELLING

Technically any psychological test is supposed to serve the purpose of a standardised measure of a sample of behaviour objectively. It is, therefore, expected that such instruments should not be biased in favour of or against any group. However, in practice, it is noticed that psychological instruments, mostly, are intrinsically susceptible to a number of sources of cultural bias. This is more so in India, as India has a heritage of multicultural scenario. Diverse etiological cultural settings—owing to linguistic, geographic, and religious variations—present a complex and constant demand on a clinician for its accurate application and interpretation. Blind borrowing of the Western tests would have dangerous consequences in pursuing diagnosis in our country. Shenoy and Kapur (1995) examined sensitivity of behavioural problem scale of the children behaviour checklist in Indian population. They reported that most of the items and cut off scores of Schenbsche and Edelbrock's are found unsuitable for use with Indian children. Several tests of the Western origin are found unsuitable for use with Indian adult population as well. Thus, discontentment has been raised by many clinicians and researchers in using psychological tests onto our population which have been developed in other cultures.

Though there is a tremendous development in publishing variety of psychological tests to suit the needs of contemporary Indian society (for detail, please refer Chattopadhyay, 2010), the concepts, however, have been borrowed, by and large, from the Western psychological literature. The self-report measures we often employ now-a-days use statements which are pertinent to Indian social set-up and thus the content is conceptualised to some extent. The problems of cultural bias, though partly, can be overcome in this way, the conceptual mapping remains problematic so far as understanding the presence of the phenomenon in the culture and its distribution are concerned (Srivastava and Misra, 1996; Srivastava, Tripathi and Misra, 1996). Many tests have been adapted onto Indian population. However, care must be taken to see that adaptation does not turnout to be mere imperfect translations of some of the tests of other culture.

Puhan (1982) in this context suggested that the conventional reliability and validity assessment should by substituted by psychometric invariance assessment which simultaneously evaluates both consistency and meaning of these tools in more relevant terms. He also suggested the necessity to fulfil the prerequisite of including many marker variables in the factor analysis of the test under consideration. Many well standardised psychological tests are differently perceived by the subjects belonging to different age, sex, religion and culture. A counsellor, particularly in India, has to be sure about such variations in test results as here we have individuals of different ethnic background.

To meet the needs of the socio-cultural tradition of India, necessity to have indigenous psychological tests have been conceptualised by many Indian scholars (e.g., Mishra, Nizamie, Shukla *et al.*, 2000; Malhotra, Malhotra and Basu, 1999; Venkatesan, 2002 a, b; Masroorjahan, Hochnizamie *et al*, 2002). Several psychological tests have been developed and adapted (e.g., Kapur, Barnabas, Reddy *et al*, 1994; Scafuza and Kuipers, 1999; Chattopadhyay, Mallick and Spielberger, 1984; Basu and Banerjee, 1998; Basu, Banerje and Mukhopadhyay, 1996) which have shown satisfactory reliability and validity as a clinical tool for assessment of the subjects of our culture.

Question may be raised about the applicability of those psychological tests which are designated as culture-free/fair; there too, our patients sometimes find it difficult to understand what is required of them while taking the tests. For example, the Raven's Progressive Matrices Test, where particularly our rural population, even though they have formal education, fail to understand the basic concept of the test designs simply by going through the instructions given in the manual. They often require further explanation. While providing further information or explanation, as the case may be, the test might lose its significance. Likewise, mere translation of the items of a given questionnaire in local language without adaptation is unscientific.

Generally it is assumed that psychological tests are devices designed and developed based on sound psychometric principles. In practice, however, all the tests available for use do not undergo such rigorous procedure (Misra, Sahoo and Puhan, 1999). Secondly, each test developed has certain basic principles. There are, for example, so many intelligence tests, but in basic principle one may differ widely from that of the other. While selecting a given test, the counsellor should have a thorough knowledge about the rationale behind the test, and also about the purpose of his/her selection in context to a given client. Selection of a test must not be done based on its mere face value only.

Psychological tests are used for different purposes (Rao, 1981). Broadly, these are useful in situations which involve prediction and acquisition of deeprooted information of the client relevant for counselling. Also, these are used for screening purposes. That is, to determine whether the client has any obvious problem for which he/she requires this type of assessment. Thirdly, the most important use of psychological tests is to understand the psychopathology behind symptoms, particularly in those cases where the client shows resistance to unreveal information. Thus, these test findings help to arrive at a diagnosis and thereby to rule out the possibilities of differential diagnoses. Fourthly, psychological tests are useful for evaluation of counselling outcome. Overall, psychological tests purport to provide an unbiased objective understanding of the clients.

A counsellor has to take a lot of precautions while selecting a psychological test and also in interpreting the test results. While selecting—

(i) the counsellor must know whethere the given test has been developed for use on normal subjects, or if it is an appropriate clinical tool.

(ii) the counsellor must be knowledgeable in deciding whether a given test can be applied for the purpose of repetitive measures, viz., pre-post design in confirming improvement after intervention.

(iii) If at all the same test can be applied repetitively, a counsellor must have adequate knowledge of time gap to be provided with between two such assessments, with a view to avoid contamination of the data due to carry—over effects.

Many a times, in practice, it is found that clients move from one counsellor to the other within a span of time and without any enquiry whether the client has been subject for psychological assessment before (if so, how long ago), the counsellor administers the same test again onto the same client which has been administered on him/her before. This is not only unscientific but unethical too.

(iv) Sometimes a given client's mental status examination demands that more than one test be administered for a particular faculty, to yield a composite picture. Test findings may appear inconsistent. But combining such different—and at times even contradictory—test results to have a comprehensive idea about the client's status requires very sophisticated training of psychometry on the part of the counsellor. Untrained personnel can never have that proficiency, adequacy, and sophistication required for reconciliation of such diverse test scores.

(v) If the client provides the counsellor with previous psychometric test results (done in a different set up), it is better to consult those only after the counsellor (with whom the client is associated now) has framed his/her own opinion about the case unbiasedly. Prior information about the previous test results may bias the counsellor about the later assessment.

If, however, the psychological assessment is done by another clinical psychologist, who does not happen to be the counsellor of the case, then also it is better that the clinical psychologists remain double-blinded in this regard.

(vi) Lots of controversies exist amongsts scientists over statistical and/or clinical interpretation of the test results. Statistical interpretation of psychological test results may ignore biological/behavioural significance of the data. Even when statistical significance is not reached, the importance of valuable data obtained on a very rare, atypcial case cannot be ignored. Interpretation of data and its clinical correlates can be determined only by a trained counsellor.

(vii) In general, it is seen that there may be chances of faking data by the clients on questionnaires/inventories. As opposed to this, some modern scientists are of the opinion that since the given test is a standardised one, the counsellor can accept the data as it is, on matter whether the client manipulates data by responding in a socially desirable manner. But this argument does not appear to be sound. If, for example, we find very high 'L' scale score for a given client on the E.P.Q. test, it is our duty to see why the client requires that degree of manipulation, instead of just accepting the score as the test is a standardised one. Maybe that the reasons for obtaining very high 'L' scale score for a given subject could be verified through objective tests, viz., projective, and psychophysiological (GSR, etc.). The very purpose of administering psychological tests is to interpret test results clinically (with a view to facilitate counselling outcome), and not to revalidate the standardisation procedure of the given test. If test results could just be accepted as scores for a given client, then administration of psychological test could be done even by non-psychologists. Needless to mention that the task of the test administrator is not merely stating the obtained scores with the provided norm, but to intrpret the scores clinically.

In sum : Choice of a psychological test for counselling purpose, depends upon—(a) the counsellor's sound knowledge about the rationale of the given test, (b) his/her objective of administering a given test, and (c) his/her expertise in interpretation of the otained test scores.

(viii) In practice, however, a counsellor with clinical professional expertise must not be test-bound. Psychological tests may be used only to supplement other available information when necessary.

(ix) A counsellor's attitude must not be to utilise psychological test scores to facilitate an instant diagnosis of the case, ignoring all other information obtained through interview. The counsellor must develop confidence in his/her own clinical acumen and psychological tests must be administered not as a rule, but as an exception. Otherwise, it might burden the client both clinically, financially, temporally, and emotionally. This could be one of the reasons for the client's frequent shift from one counsellor to the other, which is detrimental to uphold his/her psychological well-being.

(x) The counsellor must not be preoccupied only with the morbidity aspect of the client. A counsellor's attitude rather should also be to see healthy aspects of the client's potentialities, and overall personality. While administering a psychological test, a counsellor must not assume a "judgemental role" (Brammer and Shostrom, 1968) in the sense of labelling the client with a diagnosis.

To evaluate psychological status of a given client based on self-rating scales only may be subject to falsification for various reasons. Use of such scales rests mainly upon assumption that clients are always motivated to read the items carefully, to understand its meaning clearly, and to express their feelings exactly. But in practice, however, it is found that some of the clients and mostly patients show lack of motivation to read the items carefully and to fill in the questionnaire properly. In a study in this context, Suhail (2000) reported that a sizeable proportion of the Asian respondents complained about difficulties in understanding the concepts behind each of such tests. But an adequate knowledge about the client's unrevealed materials can be obtained through projective tests. Projective tests are also not free from limitations, though these tests are acclaimed to provide unlimited space for response while the meaning of the response is not transparent to the client. These tests introduce an element of subjectivism. As an example, mention may be made here of the research reports of Puhan and associates (1995), who constructed a number of tests involving a projective inventory approach. The purpose of devising such tests was to assess aggression, dependence proneness, responsibility taking behaviour, etc. They have demonstrated a low correlation of these measures with social desirability as compared to the correlation obtained between self-report measures and social desirability. But in projective tests also, interrater reliability has to be determined which again demands more expertise. Neuropsychological test methods have helped to overcome such bias (Chattopadhyay, 1998), but there, too, a counsellor must have adequate training to interpret the results.

An adequate knowledge about the autonomic vis-a-vis biological stability and central capacity for arousal modulation necessary for life adjustment can best be understood through indirect measures like EEG averaged evoked responses, blood pressure, ECG, GSR, and some such other devices, whether the experimenter is not at all dependent on the subject's verbatim reports (e.g., Mukhopadhyay, Dey Chattopadhyay *et al*, 1996; Mohanty, Das *et al*, 1993 a, b; Sanyal, Chattopadhyay and Biswas, 1998; Mukhopadhyay and Chattopadhyay, 1994, 1995, 1997 and 2000; Chakravarty, Saha and Chattopadhyay *et al*, 2001). Such measures can be utilised safely with moderate level of precaution, as repeated measures; also these data help to evaluate post-intervention outcome.

My personal research experiences with my faculty members do show that EMG for clients with functional torticolis (e.g., Mukhopadhyay, Basu, Chattopadhyay, 1994), EEG evoked response for patients with GAD (Chattopadhyay, 1983; Chattopadhyay and Biswas *et al*, 1980; Chattopadhyay, Cook, Toone *et al*, 1980) and GSR for different categories of psychiatric patients (Chattopadhyay, Bond and Lader, 1975; Chattopadhyay, 1981; Chattopadhyay and Das, 1982; Chattopadhyay, Majumdar and Basu, 1982; Chattopadhyay and Majumdar, 1982; Chattopadhyay, Dasgupta and Laha, 1982; Chattopadhyay and Biswas, 1983) can be very successfully used for both diagnostic indications as well as for therapeutic outcome. These data can be used as biological markers both for the purposes off understanding psychopathology behind symptoms, and also for evaluation of intervention outcome. Such markers have also been used by others in Indian set up (e.g., Michael, Mirza, Mukundan and Channabasavana, 1993), for the purposes mentioned.

Chapter 10

ISSUES RELATED TO THE PERSONALITY AND TRAINING OF COUNSELLOR

Personality

A professional counsellor, in clinical domain, must have adequate knowledge about his/her own self. He/she must be in a position to evaluate himself/herself in unbiased way. Such evaluation has to be done in terms of a counsellor's own strengths and weaknesses in pursuing human interaction professionally, in order to ameliorate the problems of others, prior to launching into a delicate job of a clinical counsellor. Self-evaluation is essential to ensure (oneself) that he/she is competent enough to understand and to deal with the problems of others. Two years' full time professional internship training programme enables one to ensure further whether such required qualities have been crystallised in him/her and to decide upon whether one can pursue the profession of a clinical counsellor. Mere academic qualifications are not enough to judge the reliability of his/her views about the case – both diagnostic and therapeutic. Personal qualities (mentioned earlier by Rao, 1981) and clinical acumen together determine the authenticity of his/her judgement as a counsellor. Some of the required personality qualities considered essential for an efficient clinical counsellor will now be depicted briefly.

1. Patience

The counsellor must be competent enough to unveil the inner world of the client, keeping in view the patterns of connotations of the culture which the client has imbibed. Since elicitation of the roots of the problems reported by the client is time-taking, the counsellor must have patience to—

(i) provide the client with an empathetic listening which, in turn, enables him/her to realise the nature of his/her owns problem; this, consequently, helps the counsellor to get the client motivated for further probing;

(ii) to remain undisturbed if any obstacle arises during the process of counselling;

(iii) the counsellor must not be in a hurry to react. He/she should even be prepared to receive negative comments even. For example, in marital counselling, one of the partners might feel and express that the counsellor is showing partiality, in his reaction, to the other partner. "Dr., please don't mind; you are not supporting me; I think you are favouring my husband.... " The counsellor must have patience to bear such comments so as to make it clear to the client in due course that question of such partiality does not arise. Sometimes, clients urge for immediate resolution of their problems, or immediate answers (in client-centred approach), for e.g., from the counsellors. The counsellor must not be trapped by such persuasion from the clients;

(iv) not to be overwhelmed with joy of success when noticed initial improvement of the client; not to be disappointed either;

(v) if the client takes quite some time to show indications of improvement;

(vi) to have patience to tackle intermittent problems, if any, even after the client had shown remarkable improvement initially.

2. **Farsight**

The counsellor must keep in mind that (i) at times real causes of the client's obvious problems my not be identifiable in manifest forms; (ii) also that, some seemingly innocent causes may be mistaken as his real problems. This demands a keen and farsighted observation on the part of the counsellor.

3. **Tolerance**

The counsellor should have tolerance to accept individual differences in perception of the environment; otherwise he/she can't have respect for various types of personalities; can't maintain sacredness of the client as a human being.

4. **Control**

Must have strong determination to maintain confidentiality of the secrets the counsellor is informed by the clients; under no circumstances should he/she leak out such secrets publicly. Must not be impulsive, must respect the boundary of privacy. Otherwise, counsellor can't render services to the humanity with proper responsiveness, responsibility, and dignity.

5. **Alertness**

The counsellor has to be very vigilant at all times. Though in counselling, predominant mode of communication is verbal, the counsellor must not miss non-verbal cues provided by the client during a session. Because, these may, at times, provide significant meaning about the client's problems than those expressed by the client verbally. The counsellor requires to develop a sixth sense which enables him/her to hear even the unspoken information and clinical cues. That's why, using mobile, attending telephone calls during the session is strictly prohibited. Speed of voice, distinctness in articulation, use of intonation, flow of communication, especially long pause etc. are significant cues, to the counsellor, provided by the client. An expert clinician can easily identify whether the client uses defences like projection, reaction formation, and so on. However, counselling environment must not be viewed as a 'cross-examination' situation (Dave, 1991).

6. **Emotional Maturity**

Needless to mention that, in general, the prime objective of clinical counselling is to help the client move from a state of immaturity towards a state of maturity. Emotional immaturity on the part of the counsellor can cause serious damage onto the client.

7. Responsibility

Responsibility—legal and ethical—that a counsellor has to take determines the basic theme of code of conduct of a counsellor as a professional expert. With written consent the client is to be taken up for help. The counsellor must be competent enough to provide the client with expert opinion. If, however, the counsellor feels incompetent to apply a suitable technique of counselling for a given client, he/she must refer the case to another competent consultant. The counsellor must be ready to persent himself in front of a hon'ble Magistrate in the Court of Law, if situation demands. It is the responsibility of the counsellor to maintain atmosphere in such a way that the client can keep up regards for him (but never hate). The counsellor must maintain confidentiality of the case in every respect (detailed discussion has been made earlier in this treatise).

8. Morality

Individuals have certain similar basic needs (psychological), like need for security, need for support, need for attention, love, and so on. But individual differences do exist in the perception of such needs and also in their modus operandus. These are largely determined by cultural values and norms. For example, the ultimate aim of life for every individual is happiness. But the concept of happiness and modes of obtaining it, and its extent, are, by and large, determined by the value system of the individual. The counsellor by no means should violate such social norms, with the plea that some other cultures do not have such values. The latter decision of a counsellor would in future be recognised as exploitation by the client himself/herself. This would have a detrimental impact onto the client's emotional status. It is the counsellor's obligation to rescue a client from such tendencies, like over-involvement with the counsellor during and beyond the counselling session. It is an important function on the part of the counsellor to help the client to resolve such tendencies; or else counselling in real sense of the term will lose it significance. Contrary as it might sound, the counsellor, though requires to establish an empathetic relationship with the counselee, that relationship is strictly professional in nature. Thus, the counsellor should be in a position to maintain professional distance with the clients to avoid moral boundary violation.

9. Integrity

Moral soundness and upright personality characteristics of a person have been designated as integrity by some authors (e.g., Dave, 1991).

10. Genuineness

Without authenticity and genuineness, counsellors cannot make an adequate impact of their services on their clients in clinical set-up. Obviously, non-technical, semi-technical persons must not be licensed to conduct sessions, as they are not authentic for clinical counselling. Rogers (1957) long back stated that "... you be yourself, freely and deeply..." (p. 97). If not bona fide, both legally and academically the counsellor should never exert himself/herself fully to offer such services to the client.

11. Confidence

This is essential for any profession, and counselling is no exception to it. Confidence is especially required :

(i) To establish rapport. This is a very fundamental stage in establishing official/formal working relationship with the client. This is established well only when the client can develop trust onto the counsellor regarding the latter's (a) expertise as a professional, (b) strict adherence to confidentiality, and that of (c) ethical standards. Attitude of the counsellor also plays a vital role in this regard (see attitudinal domain).

(ii) In the selection of a technique of intervention for a given client and also for its execution. Sudden change of intervention method during the process of counselling is not desired as it can cause damage to the client. Such interruption in the intervention strategy can be avoided through adequate clinical training and experience. The counsellor must be well-versed with the inclusion-exclusion criteria for a given technique and also about the basic concepts of a given technique.

(iii) To handle confrontation. Confrontation during counselling may arise from two perspectives—(a) from the counsellor's point of view, and (b) from within the client. In the former, the counsellor experiences confrontation with the client on some concepts of counselling strategy; for example, the client may not accept the concept of unconscious, though the counsellor may think that such an interpretation is required. In the latter, confrontation is apparent from within the client. The counsellor must not be disappointed by such initial disagreement with the client. Nor should it bring down in any way the counsellor's positive regard for the client. On the contrary, such controversies should provide the counsellor with further insight into the client's thoughts, images, and attitudes in an indirect manner. Such differences/discrepancies in the attitudes have been designated as "double messages" by Ivey *et al* (1997). They demand more attention for resolution. Such discrepancies would have lasting impact on the clients' realisation of their assets and limitations in a better way, for its adequate application to their life adjustment.

Case Illustration : Male 24 years, B.E., employed, unmarried, above average in intelligence, but average performance in examinations (history of failure in two semesters at B. Engg. course), has one younger brother of bright career, hails from an upper-middle class family, was referred for counselling; had consultant psychiatrists, but was irregular in taking medicine. History of heroin addiction and sporadic but excessive use of alcohol (last 4-5 yrs), so much so that he failed to maintain regular academic schedule; spends money lavishly and whimsically. High drive to complete P.G. course and to have a dignified job but lacks determination; no intimate friend, discrepancies noted in his thought and action are—(a) perceives himself as a powerful man with high level of efficiencies and potency, but lacks confidence with a feeling of inadequacy, and impotency; (b) understands that if he is motivated to study just for a few hours/day, can do much better than many others, but appears to have a need to fail; (c) ambivalent attitude toward both the parents, persons of the opposite sex and about his own orientation to sexual life style (the latter could be revealed after a few sessions of interview); had sex relations with both the same sex and opposite sex persons; though apparently wants to prove that he is heterosexual (to keep up Indian social expectation), has strong inclination towards homosexual interaction (caused guilt in him); (d) behaviourally, apparently submissive, but expressed bouts of anger and aggression during interview; outwardly well-behaved, but uses abusive language while describing his interaction with acquaintances; physically underweight, but desires to be an impressive figure. A counsellor must have insight into the dynamics of such discrepancies in behaviour and thought of the client and also have confidence to handle discrepancies with patience.

(iv) **Handling pauses :** Pauses can be utilised as cues to deep rooted emotional problems of the client. Pauses are not very unlikely during counselling interview/discussion. The client is at a lost to find exact password to express his inner mind; may be overloaded with inhibitions. The counsellor must not feel uneasy in handling such a conflicting situation. He should not insist upon the client to speak right on the spot, but to allow him to prepare himself for expression when comfortable. A meaningful gesture, understanding link, and not pointing anything in particular may help out the client to initiate talk again. Sometimes initation of some general conversation helps the client to break the silence. Also, the counsellor must be aware of the cultural norms of the client; whether that has got any relation to induce a long pause in the client. Thus, an expert clinician counsellor should have the ability to communicate through the language of silence.

12. **Attitudinal Domain**

Attitude of the counsellor plays a vital role in establishing counselling relationship. The counsellor's initial dealings must provide the client with a message (non-verbal) that it is nothing unusual to have problems and to seek assistance for it. Such an acceptance helps the client to feel free and to communicate with the counsellor his fear, guilt etc. A sense of security the client should receive from the counsellor's attitude.

(i) **Empathy**. Empathetic attitude requires that the client be accepted in totality. Totality here means that the client is an individual, who, too, is not free from his/her family and cultural traditions that have been inculcated in his/her thought. Empathy, however, would not mean that the counsellor has to give up his/her own identity in terms of beliefs, standards, and values (Rogers, 1957; Gendlin and Hendricks, 1978).

(ii) **Positive Regards**. This is close to respect and warmth. Rogers (1957) demonstrated this as a part of empathetic attitude. Positive regard means to identify, and recognise the values, strengths, and potential resources in the client, and to ensure that the client can exercise these resources, in further, in his life adjustment. Such identification helps in bringing initial changes in the client through counselling which has a long term prospect. Such a means to bring initial change has been designated "minimum change therapy" by Tayler (1961). Such an attitude to search positive aspects of the client can be fostered through different ways, namely, 'resource development' (Carkhuff, 1969), and expectations and acceptance of the problems, in 'solution oriented therapy' (O'Hanlon and Weiner-davis, 1989).

(iii) **Constructing relationship**. Client-clinician relationship is unique compared to any other relation between two individuals. Therapeutic relationship has long been designated as a 'contract' (Meninger, 1958). In this relationship both the clinician and the client learn together. The question of superiority or domination does not prevail in it. Constructing and maintaining such a relationship represent less of hierarchy, and more of equality, which has been described as 'egalitarian clinician-client' relationship by Rigazio-Digilio *et al*, (1997). Such a therapeutic alliance requires conscious monitoring on the part of the clinicians to guard against superimposition of their own perception as well as their perception of the society onto their clients. Clinician-counsellor's personal reality must not be imposed upon as truth onto the client. Such an attitude on the part of the clinician is easier to hold in client-centred approach in counselling/psychotherapy rather than the traditional psychoanalytical approach where Freud's view turns out to be the client's view. However, in context of developmental counselling framework, the clinician can, perhaps, maintain such an attitude with regard to Freudian approach too. The latter, of course, requires modified training on the part of the counsellor-clinician.

(iv) **Openness and spontaneity**. Openness, honesty and spontaneity though are central to the counselling process (Rogers, 1957), Liberman, Yalom, and Miles (1972), on the contrary, stated that "open, authentic" group leaders produced more emotional casualities when compared to conservative counsellors. The latter can develop relationship relatively slowly. However, once again, it depends upon the expertise of the counsellor as to how to develop a working relationship, on matters whether conservative or open. In Indian set-up, at times promptness and spontaneity are found to be damaging to continue session. This has been discussed in the last part of this section.

(v) **Personal Touch**. Personal touch here means an empathetic approach towards the counselling service. This, however, must not deteriorate into an emotional involvement with the client. Dave (1992) in this connection opined that "an unusual personal touch appears to ignite the spark of life in the counselling environment". In context of Indian culture, Dave (1991) further mentioned that the counsellor's personal approach "should not carry any shade of pity, compassion or sympathy". The counsellor should try to project himself/herself to the counsellee's situation, with a view to visualise the counsellee's feelings. But the counsellor "should in no way suffer, laugh or crave with him to the context of clouding his own scientific vision" (Dave, 1991) to fulfil his/her professional responsibilities.

In sum : Dedication to the profession, determination to reach the goal successfully, adequate proficiency in selecting and executing alternative means (techniques) ensure a safe reach to the goal. These are essential prerequisites for a counsellor. This is possible only when the counsellor has an attitude to develop entanglement with the mystery of the client, so much so that removing obscurity of the problem behaviour of the client becomes his/her object of contemplation.

Indian Scenario

Training : Compared to the previous years, in the last era, training facilities in clinician psychology in India has ben relatively better. Along with the pioneering institutions like NIMHANS (Bangalore) and CIP (Ranchi), training commenced at few more centres including Government Psychiatrict Hospitals (RINPAS, Ranchi), Private Medical Colleges (KMC, Manipal, Ramchandra Medical College, Chennai) and some of the private institutions like that in Secunderabad (Sweekar Academy of Rehabilitation Sciences, Secunderabad) and National Institute of Behavioural and Allied Sciences (NIBAS), Delhi, Institute of Post Graduate Studies in Psychiatry (S.S.K.M. Hoispital, Kolkata) offering M. Phil in Clinical Psychology. Recently, a course in

M. Phil (Clinical Psychology) is also being offered at the University level—namely Calcutta University--first of its kind in India.

It is unfortunate that despite the availability of such facilities in India, many untrained/semitrained personnel and some even without any basic degree in psychology are found to render counselling services, and that too, in clinical field (Prasad, 1997). It is disappointing to observe that some such educated persons also fail to understand the dignity of the profession. This shows that they have not developed the attidude required to accept clinical counselling as a prestigious technical job. If this be the situation with such counsellor(s) then perhaps it is no wonder that some of the clients may fail to understand the intricacies of this technical job. The present scenario is a warning alarm, least the clinical counselling lose its original connotation. What is indigenous in clinical psychology is a clinical attitude, which is necessary not only to learn but also to do something about it (Wyatt, 1988).

Self Disclosure

Self-disclosure—it is better to avoid self-disclosure to the extent of providing personal opinion of the counsellor in decision-making process of the client. For example, 'I would have done this had I been in your position'; or to cite examples from personal life experiences, which in turn might cause hindrance to maintaining professional distance with the client outside counselling set-up. This can be taken as a precaution, especially in Indian set-up, as, by and large, out clients are inclined to depend on the counsellor in every possible respect.

Likewise personal touch, viz., shaking hands, at the end of the session, particularly with the persons of the opposite sex is sometimes misinterpreted by the clients. On the contrary, sometimes shaking hands, particularly with shy and inhibited type of clients helps raising self-regard of the client. Such issues require adequate resolution and to be tackled with care, caution, and patience by the counsellor, considering the sub-cultural and cultural norms of the given client.

Immediacy versus Delay in revealing the truth

Desired personality qualities, including attitudes, and nature of specialised training necessary for a counsellor, in general, have been depicted above. But these require further probe in relation to our cultural set-up. The following few pages highlight the problems a counsellor usually has to face in dealing with clients in Indian scenario.

The goal of counselling is to help the client solve his/her problems at the earliest. An experienced counsellor would think of immediacy depending upon the (a) severity of the problems reported; (b) whether problems are intertwined; (c) whether some of the complaints reported are offshoot of a major problem; and (d) hierarchical need of the client to solve the problems etc. But, in India set-up, the counsellor may have to wait for quite some time to touch upon the crux of the problems. Because; for certain issues, due to cultural inhibitions, impositions, clients take lots of time to divulge the truth, though the counsellor understands the fact in the very beginning of the session. For example, problems for which the clients, particularly adolescents and young adults seek immediate attention and help from the counsellor may have its root in an altogether different domain of life, say sexual attitude and orientation of the client. Still clients feel embarrassed to discuss such issues, and if the counsellor cotinues sessions on those areas of personality, the clients feel that the session is useless and discontinue intervention. It may be wiser on the part of the counsellor to delay discussion of certain specifics, though these are very vital from the point of view of psychopathology. In the initial sessions our clients, by and large, prefer discussion on shuttle factors rather than focussing on psychopathology. Such delay enables the client to prepare himself/herself for self-disclosure. For example, cases with masturbatory guilt and those with history of illicit sex, sexual abuse etc., are found to be highly defensive in the initial sessions to discuss about matters related to sex. This is because they are afraid that discussion/confession on such matters would debar them socially (as society expects that for teenagers to be ignorant about such matters is good). If, however, the counsellor wants to focus on such incidents of the client's life, the teenagers complain to their parents that the counsellor enquired about very nasty/dirty matter. Some of the parents also feel proud to report that, though their sons/daughters are physically mature, they are totally ignorant about sex!!

Case Illustration

A student of Class XII, aged about 18 years, has one younger brother, hails from a upper-middle lass educated family, as referred for counselling with frank OCD symptoms. He was on medication for quite some time. He appeared shy and reserved during interview. Through assertive training initially he could be helped to interact with others freely. A noticeable change was observed in him in his interaction pattern with the counsellor also. Throughout interview, he was found very resistant to discuss matters related to sex, girls, etc.—so much so that he denied altogether his experience of masturbation, and even his attitude/impression about masturbation. Such a denial of the fact gave an impression to the counsellor that he has had problems related to it.

Instead of insisting him upon continuing discussion onto such matters, initially the session used to take place on the nature of conflict, impact of conflict, guilt etc. in our life, in general. After the 5th session, the counsellor felt that the client was in a dilemma whether to reveal the impact of such issues in his life. Such a guess of the counsellor was verified from the nature of the questions the client used to ask the counsellor during the session. For example, once he asked, "Well, Sir, as we have discussed such issues, is there any damaging impact of guilt in our life?" Then again, a session was taken on the impact of various guilt in our life. In the sixth session he asked questions related to the development of sexual orientation and nature and functions of sex in life. However, in the next session, the client remained absent without any prior intimation. The seventh session was devoted to development of sexual orientation in individuals in general. In the eighth session, he sought permission whether he could reveal some of his very personal life experiences to the counsellor, and expressed that he felt the urge to masturbate on the very day of worshipping the Goddess of Learning (Saraswati); tried to control it because such an act on his part—specially on such a sacred day—might cause harm to his academic achievement; finally he could not resist the urge and got involved into masturbatory act, which has caused a significant degree of guilt in him. Subsequently, he has been experiencing lack of concentration, failure of memory etc. and has developed fear of failing in the examination; later developed OCD symptoms. Thus immediacy to achieve the end result may not be applicable in such cases. However, such delay has helped to (i) keep the client motivated to continue sessions; (ii) to realise and to learn to express his inner feelings to the consultant for his own benefit; (iii) to get relief from his distress, and (iv) to achieve a relapse prevention stage.

Interestingly, when the client experienced a relief from his distress, in the end part of the counselling programme, he suddenly stated that "... well doctor, what all I have told you about may experience of masturbation on the Saraswati Puja Day, was actually a lie; I didn't have anything like that on that day". At this stage, such a defensive statement on the part of the client makes the counselling programme complicated and lengthy. Three moot questions arise which are very pertinent to decide upon the future course of counselling intervention in this case. The questions are (i) whether the client could develop trust onto the counsellor about maintaining confidentiality; (ii) sessions so far taken whether at all helped the client to resolve his conflict; and (iii) whether counselling programme so far employed has come to a stage of termination? At first impression, the answers to all the above three questions are no. The client, it shows, wanted to make himself free from such social stigma, denying the incident to the counsellor. This is alarming to the counsellor because symptoms may recur (as the client may not be firm to bold his cognitive restructuring), though he appeared to be free from his presenting complaints. Such an attempt to deceive the counsellor about the conflicts—which are culturally ingrained and require special attention—delays the termination of counselling programme.

Patience

The importance of patience as a characteristic feature of a counsellor has just been mentioned above in this section. The counsellor must have patience, even when he/she becomes aware of such deception by the client. Such an attitude of the client is, however, detrimental to maintaining the counselling process as a mutual contract, which demands that the client reveals the fact.

In Indian set-up, for example, mostly adolescents and young adults would say 'No' to those queries pertaining to their personal life events. But non-verbal cues, in such situations, provide a better meaning than their verbal statements. Thus, 'No' in their reply, in this sense, is meaningful to the counsellor considering our culture. To obviate such problem we need some objectivity in our evaluation process. Through objective measures it is possible (e.g., GSR deflections in response to certain stimuli pertaining to the personal life events of the clients) to elicit such hidden information. Information obtained through objective measures is required to confirm whether the client has been manipulating/lying in reply to the counsellor's queries. But the task remains for the counsellor to make the client accept what has been revealed through indirect measures. This, thus, takes up extra time to complete the course of counselling programme.

Objectivity

It is not exclusive to the Indian context; objectivity as a quality is required for an efficient counsellor. Objectivity at the initial stage helps the counsellor to determine, without any bias, the 'personal construct' (Kelly, 1966) of the client which are likely to have etiological significance. During counselling phase objectivity helps to establish the frames of reference for cognitive restructuring, and also to plan termination and follow-up accordingly.

Empathy and Understanding

As mentioned earlier in this chapter that the counsellor has to have an empathetic understanding. But having so is easier when the client makes the counsellor understand specific factors and the counsellor can discuss concrete specifics rather than abstracts with the client. Some of our clients prefer such openness, though mostly in India, clients do not. Thus immediacy and concreteness, as urged upon by some of the Western authors (e.g., Egan, 1994), therefore, may be employed sparingly with care, caution and from our cultural and ethical standpoints.

Openness and Spontaneity

Openness in counselling session in required to help the client to reveal his personal matters to the counsellor. Sometimes, in India, clients feel inhibited to reveal their personal matters. At times clients even state that ... "What can I say and how far I can reveal my life events to you, I don't know doctor, as because you are so senior, and you may consider me as 'bad' ...". The counsellor has to see that counselling environment provides an element of openness to the client. But to provide openness, the counsellor must not refer to his/her personal life experiences. At times clients even ask, "Doctor, what you would have done in such a situation, as I'am in now..."? The counsellor must be competent enough not to provide prompt reply citing his/her personal experiences as ready references to the client. The counsellor has to avoid such citation of personal experiences in such a way that it doesn't interrupt the counselling process. Because citation of personal reference would interrupt exercise and execution of the client's own cognitive potentialities. Moreover, in Indian set-up, openness has a negative impact onto the client. For example, if a given client narrates his guilt over some immoral act, to encourage him to overcome guilt, if the counsellor cites examples of similar events, if any, from his/her life, that destroys the respect of the client for the counsellor, instead of providing him/her a moral boost. This, in turn, brings down the positive image of the client about the counsellor, which has a detrimental effect onto the counselling process itself. The counsellor fails to maintain, thus, his/her professional responsibility.

Case Illustration

A boy of 18 was referred to a psychologist for intervention in connection with his homosexual orientation and act. The psychologist, in the first session itself, to make the client feel at ease with his current problems, cited his (counsellor's) own life experiences of similar sexual interaction. The client thereafter looked down upon the counsellor and discontinued session. He changed the counsellor and reported the same to the new consultant he sought help from.

Likewise, authenticity has to be considered in different perspective. Though authenticity is most commendable feature of the counsellor, the client may not be in a position to accept openness and authenticity. For example, in arriage counselling, in our culture, even if the counsellor, at the very initial stage, understands very well that due to deep-rooted complexes of one of the partners, the marriage turns out to be so unhappy, the counsellor may not express the fact to the couple because such openness of the counsellor will have a negative impact onto the whole counselling process. That particular partner (with deep—rooted personality complexes) would consider it as partiality on the part of the counsellor. It takes time to prepare such a client to accept his/her limitations. Of course, following inclusion criteria of marital counselling, the partners with such deep-rooted personality problems are not suitable for marital counselling in joint session together. Each is to be counselled separately for a long time. But in Indian set-up such couples mostly insist on for taking joint sessions, otherwise each become suspicious about that future outcome of counselling intervention.

Case Illustrations

(1) A medical practitioner (female), aged 26 years, accompanied by engineer husband of 33 years, came for counselling. During the first interview, the husband expressed his desire not to attend sessions as he feels, he doesn't require counselling; problem lies with his wife. So, on request from the wife, he has accompanied her—otherwise he asked his wife to report to the counsellor alone. Need for counselling for both was felt by the wife and she requested her husband to accompany her. They are married for 3 years, no child.

(2) Both the partners are engineers, age ranged between 26-30 years, married since last 2 years, no child. Both are in service. Here too, the husband was very reluctant to attend session, so much so that he did not accompany wife even for the first time while reporting to the counsellor. Wife felt the need for counselling for both of them.

In both the above-mentioned cases, on enquiry, husbands were reported to be very passive, non-assertive to their parents—particularly having strong attachment with the mother.

After a few sessions of counselling for both the cases, the counsellor also expressed the need to talk to their respective husbands. On several requests from wife, husband in both the cases did comply, and in the first case the husband came for one more day and in the second case the husband came for two days altogether, for individual sessions with the counsellor. In both the cases, same as wives, husbands too were very much eager to know the reasons for such unhappy relationship. They expected that their own perception about the causes of unhappy relation would be confirmed by the counsellor as well. But contrary to their expectations, when they were informed (the counsellor advised them several times that they need to attend sessions separately, and at that juncture it was not the right moment to discuss etiology altogether) about their personal deficits in role playing as both husbands as well as son, and that being one of the etiological factors for their present problem (they need to exert their roles in a balanced way etc.), none of these two male partners turned out for counselling in subsequent sessions. Wives further reported that their husbands perceived the attitude of the counsellor as a gesture of favouritism toward the female partners. Such a complexity occurs more, where the counsellor happens to be a person of the opposite sex. Such misperceptions also occur frequently in cases with paranoid personality. Initial individual sessions are required to help such clients to overcome their habits of colouring events/situations with their own irrational illumination. Openness—even with authenticity—doesn't work in such cases.

A second type of authenticity would be to open up an empathetic dialogue with a view to establish and maintain congruent relationship with the client. But clients show strong resistance to sit for counselling. Instead of being open to the client, if the counsellor wants to help them through indirect way, then also question arise whether such type of clients are suitable for non-directive type of intervention? Once again, it depends upon the expertise of the counsellor as to how to resolve the problem. The counsellor must decide in the initial interview session itself, the mode of counselling which will be suitable for a given client without causing any further damage to the client.

Chapter 11

PSYCHOPATHOLOGY FORMULATION

Vignette of a Case

Ms A, 25 years, engineer, employed in a corporate organisation, unmarried, hails from a traditional, orthodox Indian middle class (in socio-economic status) family, Hindu by religion, has one younger sister (college student), both the parents employed (recently mother had retired from her service) came with the complaints of—difficulty in concentration, low work energy, sleep disturbance, difficulty in interacting with office colleagues and roommates.

To start with the interview, she appeared to be in a rather depressed state. On enquiry she reported that she is away from her home town (for 12 months) on service and due to some domestic problems she is much disturbed. Also, a recent negative comment from her office boss has perturbed her so much so that her sleep is disturbed and 'mood off'. She has started thinking that she is inept and inefficient; has not had taken any medicine till date for the present complaint. No history of previous mental illness either in her or in her family reported.

Psychopathology is the systematic study of abnormal behaviour (Kleinmuntz, 1974). Every behaviour has some determinants. Psychopathology demands a scientific probe into the feelings, thoughts, and actions of the individual with a view to ascertain the determinants of his/her abnormality. It gives a wide coverage of the variations noted in the individuals's total reaction pattern, i.e., his/her personality. The concept personality represents an individual's basic and pervasive style of functioning. It arises as a consequence of the intricate interplay of biological, psychological, cultural, and environmental influences.

The impact of culture—both direct and indirect—in symptom development has been discussed in details earlier in this book (Chapter 6) and elsewhere (Chattopadhyay and Chattopadhyay, 2009). The psychological dynamics of some of the symptoms, particularly in context of Indian socio-cultural scenario, have been alluded to in depicting the gradual symptom constellaion noted in the case illustrated in the previous chapter.

Psychopathology formulation must address not only the sources but also the course of development of the symptoms. It doesn't require volumes to justify that early child-rearing attitudes and practices have negative influence onto personality development. There is evidence, for example, that frustration during oral phase of weaning may precipitate dependency striving (Yarrow, 1954), and severity of toilet training may create conflicts over excessive needs for orderliness (Wittenborn, 1956). Such a sense of perfection, if gets associated with a sense of incompleteness, may later lead to symptom development in the child. Need to be perfect along with a fear of imperfection and incompleteness causes incongruity in his/her judgement. Attention needs be given since early age of the child so that such incongruities do not get opportunities to develop. The trait characteristics just noted in the case vignette may be considered as long established patterns of behaviour exhibited as early as childhood and/or adolescence. Prolonged behavioural problems since childhood get manifested later as symptoms.

Further depth interview of Ms A did reveal that she is emotionally perturbed as her parents have recently decided to get separated. The above client has started perceiving herself as weak—both morally and psychologically. She has started feeling socially embarrassed too (smallness), due to her parents' separation. The client has also expressed feelings of helplessness and loneliness. The Adlerian concept of 'inferiority' traces an individual's inherent feelings of helplessness to his feelings of relative 'smallness' (Suinn, 1975). According to Adler, one must try to overcome such feelings of incompleteness for one's own survival, or else psychopathology is likely to develop.

In sum, personality disorders reflect those experiences encountered by children during the process of development and socialisation.

Symptoms are the resultants of many forces—forces that develop out of the interaction effects between the client's internal and external environments. Therefore, every symptom is meaningful, no matter how bizarre it might appear to others. Understanding psychopathology of symptoms is very crucial in formulating therapeutic strategy. It aims at discovering the meaning of those unusual behavioural manifestations (symptoms) in the client's life. In other words, we need to discover the basic needs of the client that are addressed through such symptom manifestations. In this sense each symptom is meaningful for the very existence of the client/patient; symptoms also sometimes help the client/patient to fight the illness (Kobb, 1973), e.g., regression.

The goals of counselling/psychotherapy vary considerably depending upon the nature of the disorder, and more particularly depending upon the nature of the symptom(s) the client reports. Symptom psychopathology is more important than diagnostic labelling of a case, for therapeutic purposes. For example, consider an individual with feelings of inadequacy. In such a case the counsellor has to find out and be sure about the social interaction pattern (including childhood interaction) of the client, which has made him/her to feel inadequate. Consequently, it may be that avoidance of social interaction has been considered by the victim as a security measure to save him/her from social humiliation

A person with trait of inadequacy, for example, may be happy when he can react more effectively (perceived by him) to his surrounding. To achieve this he would require developing, first of all adequate motivation to face the situation in his surroundings. Such readiness to take initiative and to interact adequately is possible only when he can develop self-confidence. Confidence building will help him to perceive and achieve greater reward from action taken by him rather than his long—standing habit of inaction (avoidance). Interaction will help him to learn to avoid his 'avoidance' behaviour.

Likewise, in passive-aggressive personality, the trust area of intervention would be to help the client prevent his habit of retaining ambivalence. Psychopathology formulation would help the counsellor to be sure about the nature and sources of ambivalence in a given case. Once a client can give up his habit of ambivalence he would be able to get a grip of his/her hostility (Suinn, 1975) adequately.

Individuals with paranoid ideation require an intervention strategy which can help him to overcome mistrust through developing self-trust by reducing his/her feelings of inferiority. Cognitive exercise is supposed to help such clients to recheck his/her conception of mistrust about others and also to reset his/her cognitive appraisal in a socially desired direction.

While formulating psychopathology of the case of Ms A mentioned above the following features require special mention. The client has shown somewhat negative mood, low energy, avoidance of responsibilities (due to preoccupation about her parents' separation) on first exposure to new stimuli (though attending regular routine works, viz., office assignments), high intensity reaction particularly about her roommates (felt rejected, neglected) to the extent of developing mistrust on them, feeling of rejection from her (causing insecurity led to aggression in her), uncertainty over getting any support from her sisters on demand in case she needs, sympathy towards her Mom but insecurity whether Mom would be able to provide her support if required. All these caused helplessness and loneliness in the client. Initially she was inspired by her friend to receive counselling assistance, later was found to be self-motivated to continue receiving counselling services.

During interview, initially the client appeared to be unassertive, no intertia to take challenge, a state of mind which has been described by Suinn (1975) as "low to warm up". Later, however, on encouragement, the client was found to respond positively to try new experiences; still later was found to be self-motivated to solve problems with proper clarification on etiological aspects of some of the complaints reported by her.

Due to extreme dependency onto her parents, and the fact that she has never had been away from her home town alone, her job placement outside her home town has been a strong source of stress in her. Mention may be made here that with this occupation she has got an opportunity to work in a first grade highly reputed corporate organisation. In contrast, her roommates' extraversive behaviour patterns became unbearable to her—probably as a reflection of her own inferiority concerning her parents' separation. This is so assumed because, as long as she was not aware of her parents' separation, she was pulling on well with the same roommates. Her own 'projection' of her inner inferiority might have led her to feel as if she was in a frying pan to fire situation. She decided to leave that apartment and stay alone in another apartment—such escape helped her to adjust moderately at least. Then she reported her psychological problems to her office boss, and felt little relief (perhaps her need for support got fulfilled in that way). Finally, counselling assistance helped her to regain psychological strength. So, considering her hyper-vigilant behaviour towards others' criticisms, hypersensitivity towards others reaction, and failure to role playing and also to apply adequate coping; she showed avoidance behaviour. All these probably arise from her severe feeling of inadequacy.

Major sources of stress revealed in the case

Extreme dependency of the client onto her parents throughout, but staying away from her parents; job placement for the first time in life, got placement at a super grade, highly reputed corporate organisation (name not disclosed on ethical ground); had to take the responsibility to work alone for the first time in life; compelled to interact with others for occupational requirements (basically the client is introvert), never stayed alone outside her home town, but got job placement outside her home town—that too in a Grade I cosmopolitan city. She was thus totally in a different environment, where she experienced problems related to her food habits, communication and some such other sub-cultural differences.

Basic needs revealed in the case

Need to depend on her parents; need to get support, attention and appreciation from others. Need to have nurturant and dependable partners/colleagues to ensure support and sympathy from them. Need to refrain from assuming responsibilities alone.

Psychopathology

The client has been conditioned to get consistent reward for dependency on the parents, particularly on her Mom. Never was she allowed to assume responsibilities even for the management of her personal matters. Major decisions in her life used to be taken by her parents till date. These factors have contributed to the development of attachment learning to the extent of avoidance of independent decision-making. Finally, habit had been formed to acquire constant reward from others in every sphere of her life interaction. Fear of criticism refrains her from direct involvement in taking responsibility. Because, criticism will stand in her way to get positive appraisal and attention from others (need will remain unfulfilled). Such individuals usually show reactions to frustrations in a passive way. The conflict over dependency, self-control and aggression confuse her as to whether she can fulfil responsibilities, no matter whether the responsibilities is in connection with her occupational sphere of her life or the connection with her domestic life. Dependency striving is an outcome of frustration during the oral phase of weaning (Suinn, 1975).

Such strategy that will help the client lessening her demands associated with dependency is required. Such a strategy in the long run will help the client reducing her overall anxieties, and to progress toward a more matured level of adjustment.

Considering that the above case has strong dependency personality trait, let us have a look now to the possible psychopathology formulation of dependent personality disorder in general.

Dependent personality disorder (DPD)

In 1952, the DSM-I included DPD as a sub-type of passive-aggressive personality disorder (PAPD). The trait criteria of PAPD is underlying hostility expressed through passive behaviour. namely, Sullenness and Stubbornness. The most important character trait of such individuals is the presence of contrariness between their feeling and emotional expression. Contrariness gets manifested in several ways, no matter whether such individuals are working alone or in a group. When in a group, for example, they are found to be apparently cooperative, but in the longrun they usually work poorly with others. In occupational set-up, they may support a programme in a group vocally, but turnout to be obstructionists later in their behaviour. Actually they do not have any immediate gain by causing hindrance to the progress of work, but because of their trait characteristics—viz., ineptness and procastination—they find some reason within themselves to hold back (Suinn, 1975) the work by the time other group members are ready to begin action. Thus there is enough scope for them being misinterpreted by others. It appears as though they have got a need to prevent others contributing. There initial cooperation turns out to be superficial (Suinn, 1975).

In actuality, their need is not to oppose others' progress but to attain perfection in action. Therefore, instead of taking immediate action, they focus upon having every contingencies discussed and clarified. Their endeavour for extreme perfection (out of fear of criticisms of their action by others) causes unusual delay in submission of the assigned work. The same picture prevails when they work alone. Then too, they delay so much for rectification/modification of the assigned work that deadline for submission gets expired. Their sincere endeavours to get reward from others as 'perfect workers' gets jeopardized and thus they become subject to misinterpretation by others. Such unfulfilled need induces further frustration-led aggression in them in a cycle like fashion.

In sum, contrariness evident from the above is—need to have perfection vs. inaction owing to procastination.

Contrariness as trait characteristics is evident in several ways in the life interaction pattern of such individuals. Individuals with DPD show a pervasive behaviour of extreme inability to act independently and also to expedite adequate decision making without support and directions from others. This is due to lack of confidence in them. They lack leadership qualities and show avoidance in assuming responsibilities. Such an all-pervasive inability has a detrimental impact onto their sense of individuality and self-identity, so much so that they don't perceive it as interference even if others apprehend in making decisions about their personal life matters related to their education, occupation, marriage and so on. Owing to such a severe dependency need they are found ready even to endure mistreatment by others; they can tolerate any kind of behaviour on the part of others no matter whether it is self-derogatory to them. Their ultimate gain is to maintain a dependent relationship. They can't assume positions, though longing for them, because of lack of self-assertiveness. Gray and Zide (2008), in this connection, mentioned that problems of such individuals are more than just being 'indecisive'.

In sum, contrariness here is between their longing for positions in life but not being able to assume responsibilities.

While formulating psychopathology we first need to answer as to why these individuals cling so tenaciously to others at the cost of their own individuality? The most simple answer to this question is that they have some gain out of sacrifice in their lives. What is the gain about? The nature of gain may vary from individual to individual. But most common gain found in them is the fulfilment of their need to win appreciation (Hardy, Barkham and Shapiro, 1995; Nietzel *et al*, 1998) from others. They, thus, show contradiction in their judgement in the following way : on the one hand they demand appreciation from external sources to strengthen their self-esteem, on the other they fail to represent themselves, with adequate prerequisites required to get appreciation. They fail to work independently and efficiently to decide upon matters awaiting prompt decision.

In sum, contrariness is regarding need to be appreciated versus lack of initiative to exercise requisite trait qualities which facilitate getting such appreciation from others.

They feel helpless when alone. To avoid such painful experience, these individuals do not usually disagree with others; rather subjugate their needs to those of others. At first impression such behaviour may be misinterpreted by others as being compliant to the person being dependent upon. But in the long run such dependency, particularly in occupation, causes irritation in others. Excessive demands for reassurance eventually become bother some to office colleagues and most people are driven away. This cause insult and humiliation to such persons and they perceive others as unkind in such circumstances. So their apparent behaviour to comply with is to avoid painful experience arising out of anticipation of being thrown out/left out alone.

In sum, contrariness in their behaviour is apparent through the tendency to comply with and ultimate failure to prove compliance through action (ambivalence); need to be supported which gets jeopardised out of the constant fear of being abandoned.

Incongruities in the judgement of such clients get manifested in several other ways. For example, on the one hand they lack initiative to put efforts to which reward on successful completion of a work, on the other, they can't wait for deferred pleasure (impatience). Their conflict is between need to be dependent along with a fear of being dominated (Suinn, 1975). Such contradictions in cognitive sphere arise out of covert hostility to their parents, who have been mostly dominant, rigid, demanding and unapproachable. The over behaviour of individuals with DPD is nothing but a compromise by being dependent through passivity and avoiding domination through resistance (Suinn, 1975). Such resistance gets manifested as rigidity in their life activities. Needless to mention that such tendency to compromise in life is not conductive for future attainments. While formulating psychopathology attention needs be given to such factors causing contradictions in them.

In Indian culture, mostly boys show extreme dependency onto their mothers till their adulthood. Severe conflict starts in such adults initially after assuming responsibilities in occupation and, later, after getting married. They fail to exert their respective roles of an employee, as a boss, of a son and of a husband—adequately. Particularly, in home front they become subject of irritation to their wives as they can't take decision independently without consulting their mothers, even in respect of certain matters related to their conjugal live. As they are provided with more and more support and shelter from their mothers particularly, and, in general, from their parents and other family members, such individuals feel more and more insulted and humiliated by their live partner and in-laws. Reasons behind such dependency are found in their childhood upbringing, where they have developed feelings of self-doubt, passivity, helplessness, and lack of self-confidence. Consequently they fail to perform their social role adequately when self-assertion is required. In this connection Grey and Zide (2008) mention that such individuals' social relationship are apt to be related only to those they "depend upon".

Though dependent behaviour begins at early childhood, it gets manifested during early adulthood to such an extent that it can draw the attention of others. Enquiry into psychopathology reveals that such individuals since childhood have received nurturance from others to an excessive length. Their interaction, particularly with mother/mother surrogate has been such that the attachment developed is perceived by the child as being too narrowly restricted. The child doesn't learn to exercise self-competencies. Rather, he perceives the attachment with mother as being so deeply rooted that it deters the growth of competencies in him. The child thus fails to learn to obtain reinforcement by his/her own self. If the child gets adequate amount of reinforcing stimulation, that too coming exclusively from only one source, i.e., mother (Millan, 1969), it encourages development of dependency as a personality disposition. They have had no opportunity to take responsibility even in respect of some major life circumstances/situations before. In other words, they have not had opportunities to develop self-esteem through proper execution of duties assigned to them. In Indian set-up, such individuals, during their childhood, usually get reward from their parents and others as 'sober', which make them ultimately unassertive. In this sense assertiveness is misinterpreted as rudeness. Such a notion is deterimental to the welfare of the children.

Children should be given training during upbringing about assertiveness; of course, aggressive assertive behaviour must not be encouraged. Such a temporary reward ('sober') makes such individuals unassertive. They are unable to express disagreement being preoccupied with a strong feeling that they might be recognised by others as inept. They dread asserting themselves lest their actions are misinterpreted as aggressive which, in turn, will cause resentment (fear of loss of the object, wants to depend on). Further enquiry reveals that such individuals have been brought up in well-protected safe environment and have had interaction in 'closed' surroundings; they are not mentally ready to come out from such 'close circuit' (Nietzel *et al*, 1998) environment. If forced into a so-called open environment, they usually remain inhibited and afraid that they would make mistakes that will bring rejection, which, they are sure, is forthcoming. They require constant reassurance that they are not being abandoned because if left alone, they, experience that their life force gets paralysed.

In sum, contrariness in their judgement—need to be close but fear of rejection. That's why, in case of any strong demand for taking responsibility which will bring a change in their existing interaction pattern (e.g., change of team members in occupation), they start procrastinating. Such habit of procrastination has to be tackled carefully in counselling sessions.

Features of dependence are found in other personality disorders, namely, Somatoform disorder, histrionic personality, borderline personality disorder, and also in agoraphobia. (DSM-III(R) attempted to demonstrate characteristics feature of DPD and similar others which show quite a few overlapping of symptoms (APA, 1987). The differntial assessment, therefore, has to be done very carefully as the whole process is a complicated one.

Unlike other conditions which show akinness in symptomatology with these disorders, in DPD, usually the individual has a longing to hold on to a dependent relationship at least with one main person/key person in life (change, alteration, modification in such relationship is not desired by them as it causes insecurity in them), even though they may not have a strong interaction in many (Kaplan *et al*, 1994). Fear of rejection from others may not allow such individuals to intermingle with many. That they stick to atleast one person is indicative of the fact that they feel secured having been getting the opportunities to depend. Dependency provides a strong sense of security to the individual (having DPD) that he/she will not be thrown out.

Let us examine another case

Mr. X, 28 yrs, graduate, employed, unmarried, comes from a middle class family (in socio-economic status). As far as his academic achievement is concerned, he had been

that they have lots of incongruities in their behaviour. In psychopathology formulation we need to find out the possible reasons for such incongruities. Inquiry should be made to reveal their achievement need. They are likely to have high ambition but lack initiative necessary for attainment. This causes incongruities in their judgement. So, we have found out one of the reasons for their incongruent behaviour. Care should be given to see that the client learns to implement initiative-taking behaviour. Any learning required reinforcement. As a consequence of self-derogation, he/she not only fails to obtain positive reinforcements from others, but fails to obtain the same from himself/herself also. He/she as if starts spinning a web for capturing of approval both from the self as well as from the society but finally becomes an object with no reinforcement. For such clients usually reassurance that their efforts will be rewarded acts as reinforcement. We need to see here who are the agents in the clients' life from whom the clients expected reassurance but failed to receive the same. This shows that they have dependency need at a significant level. Such dependency make them incapable to evaluate their own positive efforts; they seem to remain blind about their positive qualities. Even if they have achieved something significant in life, they attribute it to chance factors (lack of self-confidence). Things for which they have been longing so far, when achieved, then those turn out to be totally insignificant. This is because such clients have never got opportunities for enjoyment on achievement; their enjoyment has been conditional. Conditional because these clients through their upbringing process have been habituated to associate a tone of threat with their life-achievements. For example, a client reported that his parents used to say on his achieving something in life — 'don't be overwhelmed with joy on what you have already achieved, be sure that you don't become a subject of humiliation by the society in relation to your life achievements you are awaiting for'.

We need to formulate therapeutic programme which can provide him adequate self-confidence for future achievement and life-adjustment. Why do they lack self-confidence? Of all the several factors which are held responsible for not developing adequate self-confidence, one important factor is that they developed habit of brooding more about future negative outcome of their efforts (apprehension of failure). Reasons for developing such apprehension are to be determined by the concerned counsellor. They are habituated to assume so many 'ifs' and 'buts' in formulating and executing achievement plans that finally make them feel that all roads leading to the goal are full of hazards. Care needs be taken to help them to come out from such severe apprehensions. They should be trained to take a view of all the pros and cons of a plan prior to its execution, but that must not end in mere apprehension which ultimately prevents him exercising initiative taking behaviour. They procastinate actions which they are required to fulfil in order to get relief from pain of failure and apprehension (in anticipation).

On the one hand, they lack-self-help strength to take initiative and also in decision-making, on the other, they show rigidity in following the guidelines they are provided with. Though they are afraid of being censored by the public (fear of rejection), and as such prefer to lead a capsuled life, (to gain security), they start censuring the procedures they are advised upon for implementation with a few to have a better coping, thus fail to progress (out of rigidity) in therapeutic endeavour. Such rigidity is out of their contradictions between need to depend versus fear of being overpowered.

Rigidity in some cases causes a serious hindrance to the progress of the therapy. Sometimes clients develop transference to that extent that they become apprehensive of losing the interaction with the concerned clinician if the sessions get terminated. In this sense, it appears as though they have no real motivation to get rid of their problems, but to retain the problems. Such clients ordinarily prefer to change the therapist/counsellor with a hope to get in touch with many such clinicians to ensure that he/she can possess at least one such expert (in case of need), if not more. Thus the whole purpose of counselling gets jeopardized.

In some cases, there seems to prevail a need to fail. Failure is in terms of their life achievements. Further probe into pathology of such behaviour mostly reveals that they have severe guilt in relation to their personal and private matters of life. Need to fail is a self-induced punishment to compensate guilt. These needs and behaviour of the clients are to be considered seriously while formulating psychopathology. Psychopathology formulation thus helps to fix-up the therapeutic goal.

A Summary on the Psychopathology Formulation of Individuals with DPD, and those with APD : Towards A Synthesis

Heightened sensitivity toward criticisms from others, hypervigilant about being rejected; hesitant to take responsibility; tendency to avoid interactions, especially when personal efforts to take initiative are demanded; lack of confidence and low self-esteem are common to both DPD and APD. Thus, in clinical practice, these two disorders may appear indistinguishable (Gray and Zide, 2008). However, based on certain basic differences in psychopathology, in spite of such commonness in clinical picture, it may be feasible to work out differentiation for counselling/therapeutic purposes. In this sense, symptom psychopathology is more important than diagnostic labelling in setting the goal in counselling/psychotherapy. For example, individuals with DPD cling to others tenaciously (to maintain relationship), so much so that they even subdue their needs to others. They don't mind to endure mistrust in order to maintain a relationship (to fulfil dependency-need), (Grey and Zide, 2008), whilst those with APD show marked social withdrawal (in apprehension of making mistakes that will bring rejection they are sure is awaiting for). One might interpret psychopathology of these two behaviour patterns in a different perspective. Both the individuals have the same need—i.e., need to have support from others. But the one (individual with DPD), wants to retain it through action, whilst the other (individual with APD) through inaction. Such a contradiction in selecting means to reach the same goal has to be highlighted in the formulation of psychopathology so that appropriate steps can be taken for its amelioration—through counselling—to help these individuals to adopt adequate coping. Such personality characteristics, if not ameliorated, will affect adversely nearly all aspects of their lives.

People can cope with stress in many ways; also individuals have their own style of coping. Constructive coping is task-relevant action oriented coping. It involves a conscious effort to rationally evaluate one's alternatives that he/she has in hand, to exert an effort to solve the problem under reference. It thus prepares one to confront problems directly. Such direct confrontation requires relative appraisal of one's sources and natures of stress and its coping strategies. For adequate coping, in counselling the client is assisted to learn how to exert some control over harmful behaviour. It is possible only when the client can achieve required self-control.

Chapter 12

COUNSELLING PROCEDURE

Counselling process may be described as a continuum ranging from awareness of the problem on the part of the client, through discovering the client's own assets and limitations required for understanding the psychological meaning of the problems, to implementation of behavioural changes in a desired direction (goal achievement). Though counselling process, by and large, is same for problems related to different spheres of life, certain important diversities in this context need mentioning here. For example, in vocational and educational counselling, emphasis is more on the cognitive aspects of the clients, while for the clients with personal/emotional problems, counselling in psychotherapeutic model gives emphasis on the affective aspect. In general, however, the procedure employed in counselling has been mentioned by Rao, 1981; since the counselling is a continuous process, in my opinion, for easy understanding and keeping in view of the present scenario of hazards the professionals come across in counselling, the whole process may broadly be divided into the following segments :

(a) Pre-Counselling

Awareness of the nature of the problem(s), and also for its amelioration through professional psychological intervention are the main concerns here. In Indian set-up, the clients are mostly not self-motivated to receive counselling services. They are mostly accompanied by their parents/relatives. Because, clients, by and large, in particular teenagers and young adults, show strong resistance to receive such assistance with an impression that they don't have any problem for which professional consultation is required; rather they feel they have been compelled by their parents to come. Just to avoid subsequent family distress, if any, owing to non-compliance with their parents' desires, they, present themselves to the counsellor very casually.

At times, it is also found that the clients do experience severe emotional problems within, but owing to social stigma they avoid psychiatric counselling. In either case, the counsellor has to be aware (A) of the client's basic needs (N), and also of the basic sources (S) available for the fulfilment of those needs. At the same time, the counsellor has to have a clear self-evaluation of himself/herself; whether (W) he/she can act as a resource person for the given client with a view to help the client to eliminate (E) his/her problems through utilisation of his/her own (the client's own) resources (R). Sequentially the steps of pre-counselling are—A, N, S, W, E, R. In short, the counsellor, prior to implementation of any therapeutic/counselling technique, has to be prepared to provide an ANSWER that clients would expect from him/her with respect to the genesis of their problems.

The counsellor, in principle, gathers information to fulfil such initial requirements through observation (O), interview (I), and case history; supportive (S) information, if required, is gathered through psychological testing to evaluate (E) cognitive potential and also for exploration (E) of deep level emotions and feelings of the client. Sequentially it stands as—O, I, S, E, E. That is, the counsellor, by now, has understood (O! I see), the extent of the distress the clients experience and for which they require counselling intervention. Also, the counsellor can confirm by this time whether the given client is mentally prepared to receive counselling services from the given counsellor. Both the client's acceptance to receive assistance as well as the counsellor's mental readiness to implement counselling technique provide a signal to proceed for the next step.

(b) During Counselling

From therapeutic point of view this is the most vital and crucial stage. An inexperienced counsellor may face problems while counselling in a therapeutic perspective. This stage, in fact, determines the nature of relationship that may develop in future between the counsellor and counselee. Thus, this phase may best be described as a bridge which connects two personalities in a therapeutic contract, penetrating through the outer defenses shown by the counselee. The nature of relationship which is supposed to develop for therapeutic endeavour depends upon :

1. **Establishment of rapport :** Mostly learners do not know what rapport is and how rapport can be established. In general, there prevails an idea amongst the learners that a few minutes talk with the client about his identification data is enough to establish rapport. In this sense rapport turns out to be a ritual, as if, somehow to talk on some informal matters with the client for a short while no matter how mechanical it is. But that isn't really so. No doubt rapport is predominantly established through talking (interview), but true gesturs, body language, and attitude of the counsellor contribute a lot in establishing rapport. Such initial interview is also purposive, and goal directed and unstructured. Tht is why rapport is commonly called the counselling interview. Thus, rapport establishment involves a scientific process. It is not one-sided. It is based on mutual-effort, and cooperation—a relation which can't be secured by force.

What is rapport? One may quote several definitions given by different authors, the gist however, would mean—rapport is an effective relationship which aids in implementing therapeutic endeavour. Any effective relationship requires reciprocation between two parties. Here too, certain characteristics of the counsellor, namely, permissiveness (frankness, freeness), patience (persistence), faith (on own expertise to deal with the problem(s)), acceptance (i.e., the client is a human being, no matter what is the nature of the experience he/she reports), and warmth (fellow feeling) help developing reciprocation. Reciprocally, characteristics like trust (onto the competency of the counsellor and on his/her ethical sense to maintain confidentiality), respect (as a professional person), and endurance (till the intervention outcome is achieved) on the part of the client help sustaining reciprocation. The above mentioned characteristics may thus be designated as constituents of such unique relationship. Sustenance of rapport is as important as its initial establishment.

Can rapport be measured?: Perhaps the answer, in one word, is no, if one wants to measure it on any scale. Secondly, if rapport, the counsellor feels, has to be measured on a scale, then that itself is an indication that the counsellor lacks confidence in understanding whether the rapport has been established. Thirdly, if extra attention is drawn towards rapport the client can be self-conscious and the counsellor may be embarrassed and, consequently, whether rapport has already been established would deem ineffective. It no doubt encounters a significant cost in the therapeutic endeavour.

How to establish rapport*? No short-cut rule, perhaps, can be sensibly suggested; nor that the counsellor requires a handful of tricks to establish it. The counsellor however, requires to have :

> An attitude which ensures the client about his dignity and respect. Such an attitude is exceptional, which perhaps no one else but a counsellor only can possess. To ensure that dignity and respect are retained well, the clients check the following in the counsellor during initial interview :

- The counsellor is sympathetic and understanding (S)
- The counsellor allows free expression of inner feelings (A)
- The counsellor provides freedom to discuss conflicts (F)
- The counsellor encourages exploration of needs (E) without reprimanding the client.
- The counsellor helps developing trust (T)
- The counsellor created environment which yields to self-awareness (Y).

From the above it is clear that the counsellor must possess the qualities which help in establishment of rapport by providing the client a sense of **SAFETY**:

S = Stands for sympathetic understanding

A = Allows to express

F = Freedom to discuss

E = Encourages to explore

T = Trust

Y = Yields to self-awareness

Once rapport is established, the counsellor gains self-satisfaction and confidence about therapeutic relationship. He/she is already one-step ahead now in implementing therapeutic programme.

The counsellor's sensitiveness to the client's needs and the attitude and readiness to reach out to the distress of the client in understanding his/her problems are

---

* Rapport establishment is a clinical art. Though there are certain common steps to be followed while establishing rapport, the clinician has to be careful in varying his approach in establishing rapport during psychometry, particularly while testing children with disadvantaged background, or from different culture, establishment of rapport with elderly psychiatric patients etc. Elaboration is beyond the purview of this write-up.

the constituents of empathy. Empathy is the capacity to "feel into", while sympathy is to "feel with" (Rogers, 1962). Empathy, in Rogers' (1961) words, is "to sense the client's private world as if it were your own, but without ever losing the as if quality. To sense the client's anger, fear, or confusion as it were your own, yet without your own anger, fear or confusion getting bound upon it ..." Thus, Rogers emphasizses transfer or change of place. Empathy is not imitation, yet the counsellor makes clients aware that he/she understands the clients' feelings, thoughts and actions. Empathy is based on a sacred relationship.

When such a therapeutic climate is established the client feels relaxed and relieved. Relieved in the sense that he/she would not have to bear everything himself/herself. He/she has got someone to share with. This contains an element of confession. This, in turn, prepares the client for the same.

2. **Catharsis :** The term catharsis refers to a release of emotions. Experimental evidences to support Freud's theory of catharsis has been depicted well by Hokanson & Burgess (1962).

During rapport establishment if the client can experience that trust has been formed, only then does he feel encouraged and reassured to ventilating his/her complexes. Trust in rapport, thus, provides the client with an opportunity to share his/her problems with the counsellor. Such reassurance has a two-fold value : (1) it prepares the client for ventilation which ultimately provides a sense of relief to the client, and (2) It also becomes a vast source of information to the counsellor about the etiology of the problems the client faces. Thus counsellor must be capable to prepare the client for such confession of inner conflicts, confusions, and contradictions. The tools used for accomplishing these ends, by the Freudians, are free association, dream analysis, transference, and interpretation.

A word of caution in this regard requires special mention here. That is, during catharsis, clients may cry, may blame each other and argue (if some other members of the family of the client require to be present), but the counsellor has to be emotionally non-involved with the client; if some other members of the family are present with the client during a session, the counsellor must not take any one's side to oppose the other.

Secondly, soon after catharsis the client is supposed to feel relieved. Sometimes he might think, though wrongly, that he does no more require consultation. This has to be guarded with adequate information to the client that catharsis is a means to reach the goal of counselling, catharsis as such is not the goal. The clients do require indepth explanation of the information cathected.

3. **Analysis :** Analysis refers to the process whereby the counsellor helps the client understand the meaning of symptoms. No symptom is accidental. In this sense, even a most undisciplined cognitive meandering of a client have psychological significance. Each statement, even images expressed through catharsis, can be related in meaningful ways to preceding ones, and, in turn, is influenced by prior thinking ("apperceptive mass", Bellack, 1972) and feelings. Since catharsis provides valuable clues about a client's significant wishes and impulses that were repressed during the developmental period, an analysis of the client's total personality is possible now. Since the roots of symptoms are found in early childhood (in this regard there is convergence amongst theoreticians though they believe in diverse views, viz., psychoanalysts, behaviourists). May be that terminology they use differs, e.g., anal fixa-

tion, conditioning during toilet training phase, etc., but the main focus is on childhood experience—the place to begin searching for them is there.

For example, a female, 23 years, graduate in technology, elder of 2 sisters, no brother, unmarried, in service, both parents alive—came with the complaints of sudden impulses for excessive food intake (even though realises well that she is not at all hungry), lack of concentration, low mood, sleep disturbance (intermittent sleep), discomfort in maintaining interaction with office colleagues, loneliness, need to cry; cessation of menstrual cycle was also reported. All persisting for 2 weeks.

She was staying in a private house as a paying guest on service ground. She was motivated to receive counselling services being inspired by her best friend who was away from the client. During counselling the client appeared to be apprehensive (whether confidentiality would be maintained strictly), emotional while narrating her problems (weeping) so much so that many a times she had to be allowed to take pause. Gradually, though, became relatively more free to narrate her problems, was found to be highly resistant many a times during interview. Taking pause, changing topics of discussion during interview, etc. provided sufficient cues to the counsellor for further probing into those spheres of her life.

Several case vignettes and interview contents have been mentioned in this chapter. This is to provide a guideline to the students as to how to analyse and synthesise the elicited information for counselling process with a clinical orientation.

Of course, clinicians come across resistance from the client while revealing their concerns uncensored. Also, even when in fact there are lots of repressed information as may be obvious to the counsellor; which requires unveiling in order to help the client understand the meaning of his/her symptoms. Such resistance, once again, requires analysis.

4. **Synthesis :** Two major functions of counselling are—analysis and synthesis. When information elicited/gathered have been analysed part by part, the next stage awaiting is synthesis. That is, to synthesise the parts into a whole with a view to make the client psychologically competent. Synthesis thus depends on the process of integration. So far diffused emotional feelings, contradictions and confusions have been analysed by the client with the help of the counsellor; that is, the counsellor has helped the client to see each of his/her feelings in its own perspective. The client also has learnt not to be unduly afraid of facing life events; he had prepared himself/herself not to withdraw, but to be concerned with those events in life which call for his/her attention. Cognitive exercises involved in the process of integration are—assimilation and transformation. Transformation here refers to attributing meaning to life events and situations in a manner which is free from fictional notions; has developed adequate orientation to face reality when confronted by it.

In fact, reframing cognitive construct and attributing a modified meaning to it requires interpretation of both the processes in reality context. The term 'interpretation' in psychoanalytic therapy has a different connotation. It refers to the process whereby the therapist helps the patient understand the transference relationship. If situation demands, however, such effort has to be exerted by the counsellor in helping the client understand the meaning of such (transference) relationship. Unless that is done, the counselling process not only remains incomplete, but also becomes dangerous, as it is likely to cause serious problems in the client in future. Some authors are of the opinion that transference relationship may not necessarily be set up in each type of therapy. For example, behaviour therapists mostly view that such relationship doesn't take place in this type of therapeutic process. But such a view does not seem to be correct. Because, in any therapeutic intervention, where therapists/counsellors' personality provides the patient/client a ground to develop security, acceptance, and belongingness (be it direct verbal interaction like psychoanalytic therapy, non-directive approach like that of Rogers, or predominantly interaction through instruments etc. as in behaviour therapy), a transference relationship is bound to occur.

Whatever may be the degree of professional and social distance the therapist/counsellor maintains (obviously such relationship must be very well-concerned with ethical issues of boundary violation), a sort of dependency, particularly in Indian culture, develops on the therapist/counsellor. Needless to mention that the therapist/counsellor must guard against reciprocating the patient/client's feelings. To make such intervention strategy a successful one, the therapist/counsellor has to take necessary steps to (a) help the patient/client understand his motivation and personality as to why he seeks such a relationship in a therapeutic regime, and (b) to help him overcome such need to become an independent, responsible, and fully functioning individual.

5. **Time schedule :** The term time here has different connotations—(i) There must be a time schedule for each session. This schedule must not vary from one client to other, so as to avoid its further negative consequences onto the counselling relationship. On an average about 45 minutes is required for each session to wind-up. Of course, it might get extended in some special cases, namely, joint session with both the husband and wife in marital counselling, (ii) time also indicates bridging the time lapsed between the past and the present life events of the client. Such a bridging obviously helps the client to build a time budget for his/her future life plan in terms of his planning and execution; (iii) time of termination when; (i) and (ii) have been accomplished, the client is expected to be ready to accept termination. Sudden termination is dangerous and must not be done. The counsellor has to provide information about termination in an appropriate time during the course of the counselling that the process has to come to an end. Sometimes some hint of termination causes turmoil in the client. The counsellor's expertise will surely help him/her to find a suitable time in connection with a given client as to when and how the client be provided with information about termination. Subsequent to formal termination follow-up sessions may be arranged.

Termination : Termination may be viewed from two angles, viz., (i) termination of each individual session; and (ii) termination of the counselling process itself with respect to a given client.

Termination of each individual session : The counsellor has to take care of the following when each session comes to an end so that the client can feel that

(i) The time spent was worth
(ii) That he has achieved something in this session
(iii) The client feels confident and mentally prepared to come for the next session.

The termination must not be abrupt. In the initial session when a time frame is given to the client about each session, the counsellor must be alert about time factor. A few minutes prior to the end, the counsellor should wind up the matter which will give an indication to the client that the session will end shortly. Homework assignment, if any, can be given after winding-up the matter of discussion, and just before the client leaves the counselling room.

The counsellor should be careful not to snap at some countinuing trend of thought of the session. If the client wants to express something before he/she leaves, or wants to clarify his/her doubts, if it is related to the matter of that session, he/she may be allowed to express it. If however, the client poses a new trend of thought (a new issue), the counsellor has to be tactful (time factor) and to assure him to take up the matter later.

Some of the clients, particularly those with dependent personality type, may want to linger the session. This should not be encouraged. An expert counsellor must know-how to discourage it and why.

Date and time for the next appointment be fixed up, with a view to have a clear idea about intervening time between two session.

Termination of the counselling process : Termination must not be abrupt. This might cause emotional problem in the client. During the counselling process the counsellor should give an information about termination to the client. Since number of sessions can vary from client to client, depending upon the number of sessions required, and progress attained in counselling (in terms of the client's maturity and self-management), the client be provided with information about termination, by the counsellor. It must not give a feeling of termination of human relations, but every individual session should ideally make the client free from counselling dependency.

Through counselling the client can change his/her attitude. Change of attitude

- is evident as the client starts perceiving things in a more rational and practical way. Such change in perception
- can broaden the client's outlook. Such a broadening of outlook
- enables the client to develop maturity. Maturity helps the
- client to develop self-acceptance (independence). Self-acceptance helps to
- come out from dependency onto the counsellor
- the client learns to accept the relationship as a professional official contractual counsellor-counselee relationship
- acceptance of such a relationship does not give a feeling of departure in the client (during termination). Rather it gives a sense of achievement in the client.

In sum : Counselling aims to change the client's outlook both internally and externally. Such broadening of outlook has to be done very carefully and skilfully. This is possible only through the attributes possessed by a qualified, trained, professional clinician-counsellor.

It is desired that the client should not fail to report to the counsellor during follow-up sessions, be it short-term or long-term, as plane by the counsellor. This would help the client reach a relapse free state on time.

6. **Insight :** Counselling helps the client gain insight into his/her problems. For example, in psychoanalytically oriented counselling insight means to make the client aware of his/her conflicts, repressions, inhibitions and also that when these are seen in their true perspective, they don't cause pain in the client.

Insight may be intellectual and/or emotional (Ellis, 1962). An intellectual insight is a necessary condition for emotional insight. Counselling, particularly, long term, depth counselling aims at providing the client with emotional insight. Adequate insight development marks the termination of counselling in real sense of the term.

(c) Post Counselling

(i) **New orientation :** Changes in feelings developed through counselling are accepted by the client. Trust has developed in him. Self-actualisation has taken place. He/She is now a fully functioning person with a new orientation and meaning in life.

(ii) **Gain :** Gain is what we mean by successful end of counselling. It is expected that the client is now able to adjust himself/herself to his/her surrounding realities making use of benefits he/she has gained out of counselling services. Thus, post counselling phase comprises of new orientation and gain.

In sum : Counselling procedure, its termination and follow-up comprise of :

- Rapport Establishment (RE)
- Catharsis (C)
- Analysis (A)
- Synthesis (S)
- Time (T)
- Insight (I)
- New orientation (N)
- Gain (G).

Counselling procedure aims at **RECASTING** the client's orientation to avoid any future split in his/her cognitive and affective domains of life.

Counselling is time taking process

As the ultimate goal of counselling is to help the client understand himself/herself clearly, it cannot be rushed. Personality is a complex phenomenon. It takes time for the counsellor to make the client accept his/her inner needs and desires and thereby to change his/her own perception and value-systems. The client may understand his/her problems intellectually, still may take time to overcome his/her resistances and to accept a modified style of life. The counsellor helps the client in taking decision rather than dictating or directing the course of action. Therefore, counselling cannot proceed at a quick pace.

Counselling is a continuous process

The aim of counselling is bidimensional. In one direction it aims to help the client solve the immediate problem(s), and in another direction it aims to equip the client to exercise his/her problem solving capacities so that he/she could be self supportive in future. Such a process with a long term future implies its continuity.

Counselling is a decision-making process

A clinician counsellor aims at helping the client in developing better insight into his/her problems, and also about himself/herself. The counselee develops abilities for analysing his/her own behaviour and learns to resume grater responsibilities, and adequate decision making.

CATHARSIS

1st Session

Counsellor	Ms K, what do you think are, in general, the causes of sleep disturbances and lack of concentration?
Client	I think, doctor, distraction.
Counsellor	Well, could you please highlight on possible sources of distraction in you?
Client	Not exactly.
Counsellor	OK, not to worry.
	Where do you stay here in Kolkata?
Client	In a paying guest arrangement, near to my office.
Counsellor	Could you please detail more about the place you stay here?
Client	Well, it's a big furnished room, shared by 2 other girls including a kitchen and a drawing room.
Counsellor	Are those two girls known to you?
Client	My office colleagues; not otherwise known.
Counsellor	How interactive are they?
Client	Very interactive between themselves, but not with me (maintain distance with me).
Counsellor	Any reason that they maintain distance with you?
Client	May be because I am of a different type, do not like their way of interaction.
Counsellor	Could you please mention one or to examples of their ways of interaction?
Client	They talk loudly; mostly about TV serials, films, boyfriends, etc.. And doctor, one of those two girls is getting married shortly. They are busy with shopping, and always talks about marriage, only. I don't find topics that I could discuss with them.
Counsellor	Miss K, if you don't mind, do you not like talking about marriage, boyfriends etc.? or do you think that you have any specific reason that you can't participate in that discussion?
Client	I fee they ***underestimate*** me; when they talk in another room (ante-room), I feel they ***refer*** to me.
Counsellor	Could you please explain what you mean by 'refer to me'?
Client	Well! They talk about me and my life style.
Counsellor	Do you think your life style is in any way different from others that this can be a subject of their discussion?

Client — My present life circumstances make me feel... (the client starts weeping)

The session had to stop here helping the client to summarise the session by herself. Home work was assignment to her on the issue of 'refer me'.

2nd Session

Counsellor — How did you spend these days?

Client — A mixed picture.

Counsellor — Any reasons for viewing it as 'mixed'?

Client — Yes, of course.

Counsellor — Could you please detail?

Client — After discussing with you, better I should say, providing you with so much of my life information, I felt relaxed, fresh, initially for two days. Later I started feeling low.

Counsellor — Doesn't matter, we shall discuss again the reasons for your feeling low.

By the way, Ms K, have you done the home work assigned to you?

Client — Doctor, I forgot to do it. Sorry (resistance?).

Counsellor — O.K. No need to feel sorry.

I'm sure, you will be able to brief me about our discussions that took place in the last session.

Client — Well, I remember certain things, but scattered again.

Counsellor — O.K. please brief me what all you remember, doesn't matter even if it is scattered.

Client — Briefed with a few lapses and gaps.

Counsellor — Well, you have briefed well with a few lapses and gaps; however, can you try to remember now some such gaps?

Client — I presume, I mentioned about my roommates ***under-estimating*** and ***referring*** me.

Counsellor — That's right.

Let's start today's discussion on underestimation and reference.

Can you tell me what is underestimation?

Client — I can try doctor.

Counsellor — Please.

Client — Considering inferior.

Counsellor — Good. Your explanation is logical.

Counsellor — Could you please explain what makes one ***think of others as inferior***?

Client	May be that one feels himself superior.
Counsellor	I'm sure you will be able to explain what makes one ***feel inferior about oneself***.
Client	When one thinks he has somehow failed to maintain social/moral norms in life interaction.
Counsellor	Do you see any such matters in your life?
Client	Yes, there are some.
Counsellor	Ms K, with such a good clarity of thought, could you please see what makes one to feel that he is being referred by others?
Client	I think it is the other side of the coin of feeling inferior.
Counsellor	Lets see now, when someone thinks that he is being referred to, and if it is a reflection of his basic inferiority, then, how can others known that Mr. X has got inferiority, and start referring to him?
Client	Doctor, I haven't understood you question (is it that the client is seeking pace?).
Counsellor	OK, I shall repeat (the question was repeated).
Client	I'm not sure doctor, whether I can answer your question (is the client seekings pace again?).
Counsellor	Doesn't matter, even if you can't, please try. I'm sure you will be.
Client	Could be that the person, because of his own inferiority starts thinking that others know about it, and talk about it?
Counsellor	Good, you have been able to answer. Then, does it mean that the person who feels inferior is conscious about the reasons for feeling inferior?
Client	Seems so.
Counsellor	Ms K, then do you think, that your roommates didn't think you inferior, you might have projected your views about yourself onto them?
Client	After a long ***pause—may be ... the client starts weeping.*** Session couldn't be continued (the client washed her face and went out).

3rd Session

Client	Appeared disturbed, with a gloomy face.
Counsellor	How are things going on?
Client	Not well, doctor.
Counsellor	Any reason?
Client	Yes, there may be, but I can't really explain to you all ***(resistance?)***.
Counsellor	Ms K, I have not requested you to explain it really. Can you just mention a few of those reasons?

Client	***Pause ...*** I'm confused.
Counsellor	Do not worry, take your time.
Client	By the way, Dr., in the last session I told you that a person is conscious about the reasons for which he/she feels inferior. But I can't relate everything accordingly in my life.
Counsellor	Ms K, there may be reasons for such apparent inability to relate everything in one's life.
Client	Doctor, whatever I say, you seem to enquire justification for that. Why is that?
Counsellor	Ms K, you are a student of science. Do you believe in the principle of causality?
Client	Yes, I do.
Counsellor	Then, do you think that my attempt to justify everything rationally is unjustified?
Client	Pause ... ***(perhaps in dilemma whether to disclose everything to the counsellor)***
	Ya! You seem to be justified.
Counsellor	Lets see now, how certain events in your life can be related.
Client	Doctor, I'm very much distressed; please help me. ***(Eyes start tearing ...)***
Counsellor	You said you are very much in distress; could you please tell me the extent of such distress?
Client	Pause... no reply for a considerable period of time.
Counsellor	Let me give you some hints. Does it disturb your sleep? Do you have adequate appetite? Do you get adequate work energy? and so on.
Client	I go to office regularly, and work whatever is assigned to me. I have, in fact, informed my immediate supervisor about my problem in concentration.
Counsellor	What is his reaction to it?
Client	He is cooperative.
Counsellor	What about your appetite?
Client	Doctor, again there is a problem.
Counsellor	Please state it.
Client	I used to take food with two of my roommates. We three used to cook in our room. Suddenly last week they have told me to arrange my food on my own. I felt very disappointed; I don't know why the ***reject*** me (weeping).

Counsellor	What you doing now about your food?
Client	I take food from my office canteen. I stay late in office, finish dinner, then go back to my place.
Counsellor	Ms K, I wanted to know whether your appetite is OK.
Client	Yes, it's OK. Rather I eat voraciously sometimes as I stated earlier.
Counsellor	Do you know why I am asking you this questions?
Client	Not really.
Counsellor	If you feel so much disturbed that you can't sleep etc.—better to take little medicine—of course along with medicine counselling can be continued.
Client	Why do you want me to take medicine?
Counsellor	Because you had reported that your mood remains off the entire day, so much so that you don't enjoy your work; sometimes you don't even like to go for a movie.
Client	No doctor, I wouldn't like to take medicine.
Counsellor	Any specific reasons for?
Client	Yes, some of my relatives had bitter experience with medication.
Counsellor	Its not necessarily true that medicine always will have hazardous effects. There might have been some other reasons, for medicine not working properly, say e.g., irregularity in taking medicine.
Client	Doctor, I don't want it. Can you not help me without medicine?
Counsellor	Well, it depends upon you. One thing I can tell you that to get the effect of counselling you require to have patience, because counselling doesn't provide you instant relief, results.
Client	I will bear it. You know, doctor I have so many problems. Please help me. Starts weeping.
Counsellor	Ms K, it appears that you are not in a mood to discuss any further today. Could you please keep in mind that—you felt ***rejected*** when your roommates arranged for their dinner separately (leaving you alone). What makes one feel rejected? We shall discuss it in the next session; so far you please try to work out on this issue of ***rejection***.

4th Session

Client	Soon after entering the room the client said, sorry doctor I couldn't workout home work.
Counsellor	OK. But any specific reasons for this?
Client	Doctor I have got so many problems, for which I need your help. But I see that instead of you telling me the reasons for my prob-

	lems, you on the contrary want me to find the reasons. Doctor how can I find the reasons? (Resistance?)
Counsellor	Ms. K, you are right, but I have noticed that, so far, you have been very good in finding some of the reasons for your problems. So, I hope that you will be able to find the answers for rest of the questions as well. Secondly, don't you think that instead of I telling you the reasons, if you can find those for yourself, that would give you a better and quicker outcome? I would appreciate it if you tell me your opinion in this regard.
Client	Seems logical. Its important what you said. I have understood what you mean to say, but can I really find the reasons?
Counsellor	No harm in trying. Please try and that way you will help me to help you. As you said before that you have come to take help from me, in this way, can you not reach your goal?
Client	I presume so.
Counsellor	Then am I not helping you?
Client	I understand your methods of helping me. But doctor I have got a question.
Counsellor	Please tell me.
Client	May be that I'm not aware of many such reasons.
Counsellor	What you mean by 'not aware'?
Client	I mean, some of the reasons may be at subconscious level. Two important implications of the client's using the term subconscious— (i) The client wants to escape disclosing even those which are at the conscious level (ii) It provides a clue to probe into subconscious/unconscious matters.
Counsellor	It sounds very logical. But what do you mean by subconscious?
Client	Let me explain in my own way.
Counsellor	OK. Before we probe into the matter in your subconscious, could you please see some of the reasons for the problems about which you are very much conscious?
Client	Long silence : Eyes full of tears.
Counsellor	Ms. K, by now you have understood that everything is very confidential here. Also, counsellor expects your free expression without any hesitation.
Client	Doctor for about last 6 months I am under severe distress, in addition to what all situational events I have already reported to you so far.
Counsellor	I see! Could you please enlighten me about your severe distress.

Client	This is centering around my parents.
Counsellor	What is it about?
Client	My parents are going to be separated : My father has already left our house, my mother is alone there mostly. Because my sister goes to her class in the morning and comes back in the evening.
Counsellor	Is it a sudden decision between your parents?
Client	Not really. We have heard that my father had had someone in his life beside my mother. My mother used to express her aggression towards my father several times before. Now my father has threatened my mother that he will go to the court.
Counsellor	What is your mother's reaction at present?
Client	She is more concerned with the shame of it all, and thinking of our relatives and friends. Also she is worried about our future.
Counsellor	Where does your mother stay now?
Client	We have a 2-roomed flat, 50% of which is of my mother's share. I'm out of station now for my service. I have got lot of things to do for my home.
Counsellor	O.K. You can do it serially on priority basis.
Client	How can I? Because, I'm not getting leave now. Secondly, I talk to my Mum only over phone. I don't phone my Dad.
Counsellor	Any particular reason for that?
Client	I was very attached to my father. He used to enquire about me every now and then. But I don't understand, how can he forget me and my sister also at this age? Does he not think about my future?
Counsellor	Have you thought of telephoning your Dad?
Client	He doesn't tell me anything about their separation. Sometimes he has disconnected his mobile (excuse!) saying that he is busy in office.
Counsellor	When you talk to your Mom over phone, what does she expect from you now?
Client	She too, doesn't want to tell me everything over phone, thinking that I will be worried. While talking, once in a while I get some such information from her.
Counsellor	What are the duties you have right now to finish up in this regard?
Client	I have to consult a legal practitioner for their marital separation. Doctor, you know, we come from a conservative family. So, my parents do not like us selecting our life partners. But my sister has selected one, I know. Now, if my Mom knows it, she will be further disappointed.
Counsellor	Do you think that your talking with parents in person back home would be more profitable than advising them over the phone?

Client	No, I won't go home now.
Counsellor	Any reason in particular?
Client	If I meet my dad, I don't know what would be his reaction. Nor do I know, where is he now. Secondly, I don't know my younger sister's stand about her future. Nor I'm sure whether she would like my intervening in her personal matter. Thirdly, I don't know my mother's reaction about my sister's decision, and also whether it is the right time for not discussing all these matters with my Mom?
Counsellor	Ms. K, these are, after all, now-a-days, not that sensitive matter that you can't face them.
Client	I have already told you that my family is conservative; I too didn't do anything for which my parents might get hurt.
Counsellor	OK, if you think that is justified, nothing to worry about.
Client	In my housing complex there is a neighbour who seemed to have an eye on me. But I have never encouraged it. But last time when I had been to my home, I found him somehow indifferent. Though I have never had anything in my mind, I feel now, you know, he might ignore me.

This might have some clinical implications to the counsellor :

(i) Where any guilt for the client for ignoring him?

(ii) Whether wanted to kill time and see the reaction of the guy (uncertainty)?

(iii) Whether the clinet used to feel proud within (that someone is after her), but never expressed?

(iv) Whether the client feels rejected now (insecurity)?

(v) Whether feeling of helplessness is present in her as from every corner she is feeling rejected?

(vi) May be not really interested in the guy.

Analysis

Inferiority : Inferiority originates from a feeling of incompleteness. Incompleteness my be in context to various pursuits at different stages of life, may be due to failure in maintaining moral standards (as in this case), or failure to be perfect (in one's life attainment), and so on. Such incompleteness makes the person feel weak; he starts feeling small. Smallness, in turn, gets related to helplessness.

Adlerian concept of inferiority, thus, traces man's inherent feelings of helplessness to his feelings of relative smallness. In the case cited above—because of parents' separation the client has started perceiving herself as psychologically and morally weak (that is small); also feeling socially embarrassed (smallness). Associated with it is her feeling of being lonely helpless and hopeless.

In sum, psychopathology of feeling of inferiority may be depicted as— helplessness related to smallness; and (ii) a sense of incompleteness/imperfection. As a sense of incompleteness it is present in the given case.

One must try to overcome this feeling of helpnessness to for the sake of survival otherwise psychopathology is likely to develop.

Resistance : Resistance, as is known, is a restraining force within the client to avoid further probe. Such probing will cause the client to experience severe threat within. So he/she manoeuvres to protect himself/herself from such feelings of threat; threat of having to face his/her conflicts during counselling. Resistance thus serves as a defense mechanism. The client seeks such defense against anxiety that could be aroused by a threatening self-knowledge of some disowned, disavowed feelings and impulses. Resistance represents an unconscious effort to avoid facing such unpleasant memories. Though counselling, particularly that with psychodynamic orientation, requires to bring to the patient's attention a recognition of such repressed memories, care must be taken, particularly at the initial stage of counselling, not to probe too rapidly and too deeply into such matters. This is to save the client/patient from further damage which might cause in him/her by arousing severe threat—through the process of revealing his/her uncounscious matters. Nevertheless, the dynamic significance of resistance during interview or intervention cannot be denied. However, degree of resistance to Its emergence and severity of implementing defensive measures are likely to vary between patients/clients.

Resistance has some positive implications too. For example, sudden shift of topic during conversation, provides a clue to the counsellor that the nucleus of the conflict is tapped. It thus provides further clues as to which are the areas that require deep level probing and also how to probe. Thirdly, it implies that the client has lots of conflicts, contradictions and confusions pertaining to that context. Though the client seeks help to solve his/her problem(s), such resistance is an apparent contradiction, as if the client is reluctant to confront his/her real problem(s). It is the task of the counsellor to help the client overcome such contradictions and to make him/her ready to confront the same.

There are various forms of resistance. A detailed discussion of it has been provided by Sandler *et al* (1970). Following Sandler and co-workers this may briefly be designated as—

(1) **depression-resistance :** Such resistance arises out of feelings of unhappiness. Unhappiness arises because the individual doesn't want to face the situation consciously, as it is painful. Therefore, such resistance emerges when the client wants to escape conscious distress arising out of some memories, and feelings;

(2) **transference resistance :** As the name implies, such resistance occurs when the client struggles against revealing his/her inner thoughts and feelings regarding the counsellor;

(3) **resistance related to secondary gain :** Indirect advantage of an illness is referred to as secondary gain. This is an attempt to suppress the 'gain' or 'value' of illness (Sandler *et al*, 1970). Usually it is a resistance not to dis-

close advantages of the illness (mostly, seeking attention, satisfying 'masochistic' trends). Resistance against giving-up well established character traits which sometimes have been perceived as resource for maintaining his/her meaningful existence;

(4) **Id resistance :** Unwillingness to change well established behavioural patterns which are derived from basic drives, like that of Id drive (aggressive drives, sexual drives);

(5) **superego resistance :** During counselling, particularly in that with psychoanalytic orientation, the client starts experiencing guilt (sexual or the like) which delays the execution of analysis;

(6) **detachment resistance :** As the counselling progresses and approaches its ending, fear of detachment from the counsellor may cause resistance.

Rejection

It is known that parental rejection during childhood is mostly experienced in the form of—lack of mothering parental negligence, child abuse, separation from parents, particularly the mother, especially with no adequate surrogate, death of parents, abandonment by the mother and so on. Feeling of rejection at an early age causes varieties of behavioural problems later.

The case under reference (Vignette I) though has not reported any such traumatic experience during her childhood, she has had a feeling of negligency particularly from her 'dad' as because between parents' interaction was not congenial; she had a strong desire to get more attention from her 'dad' but he had failed to even realise it. Though well nourished by her mom, lack of her 'dad's' closeness with her, generated in her a feeling of incompleteness.

The client has been totally dependent upon her parents even for her future establishment, namely, marriage. According to the client... "I expected full support and cooperation from my parents even for my future life plan, i.e., my marriage. I think my parents have failed to fulfil their duty completely" ... "I wonder, how at this age of their life, they could be that concerned about themselves only, forgetting about their children's future." (feeling of rejection and negligency).

Mention may be made here that in India such expectation that parents will take the sole responsibility for arranging their son's/daughter's marriage is not unusual, particularly for those who come from traditional, orthodox families, and also for those boys/girls who have been complying with and want to comply in future with their parents' expectations and family norms. For the case under reference, parents, particularly dad's, remaining unconcerned about her future had put the client in severe distress—namely, lack of security, emotional instability and other adjustment reactions to that extent that the client got mentally ready to receive psychiatric consultation. The client had started contemplating onto parents' attitude towards her—as was revealed in the end of the fourth session.

The contents of the dilemmas expressed and insecurity of the client revealed during the interview may be analysed in the following way :

No.	Prior to her parents' separation	After her parents separated
(1)	The client did not show any gesture indicating of her liking to the next door neighbour; she was not totally unconcerned either about the matter.	She has started feeling that the man may ignore her now. This shows that the mental strength of the client which she has had owing to her parents' full support and concern regarding her life settlement (marriage) and regular life activities, which has now declined significantly so much so that she wants to see someone as her standby (in her support); the question of her not liking such affairs seem to have lost its significance to her now. Because her prime need now is need for a support.
(2)	She was not that concerned about the impact of her indifferent attitude towards her neighbour.	Now when she is totally lacking any support from any corner, her previous attitude might have caused a feeling of insecurity leading to guilt in her, thinking that she did not appreciate it when she had got the attention and if situation arises, she may even be deprived of such a support from the man, at least as a neighbour, (though may not be as a life partner). Could be that her own feeling of rejection towards that man is getting projected now that she may be rejected by the man.
(3)	The client might have a sense of pride keeping the man in total uncertainty (not showing any positive gesture of her liking to the man) with an expectation that even if she was remaining indifferent, the man will remain interested in her (attention seeking tendency).	Now that she has got a feeling of total vacuum, she has been experiencing insecurity in receiving attention from any corner. Perhaps a sense of loss is working in her now. Loss not only from the point of view of her parents' support, but also in getting it from other sources, viz., the neighbour.
(4)	May be that the client did not like the man at all; also did not have the guts to express her unwillingness to him directly (Adult passivity?).	Now that she is feeling weak mentally due to absence of parents' full concern about her, she may be afraid thinking that she is helpless, won't be able to face if the man starts taking revenge onto her regarding her non-compliance (apprehension of harm, suspicion?).
(5)	May be that the client had an ambivalent attitude towards the man. Considering her own weakness (not taking initiative in getting involved) and lack of self-control (as remained away	Now that her parents got separated at this age, she perhaps has started strengthening her positive attention towards the man thinking that if parents can break their cultural norms at such an age, then what's wrong with her if she too breaks her fam-

Contd.

No.	Prior to her parents' separation	After her parents separated
	from), she created a huge barrier in her (not to get involved) and cited examples of family conservativeness and cultural barrier.	ily tradition and cultural norms by selecting a man of her own choice? But her basic passivity (in taking initiative) now is being perceived as a very strong barrier on her part as she did not reciprocate in any way to the man's initial gestures towards her. So, once again, the client's feeling of rejection is an outcome of her very severe insecurity. The man might represent now as a supportive male figure (father?) to the client, at least in the context of her social and mental security. Representation of a father figure she barely needs, but she is totally uncertain whether she can have such a supportive figure at all in her life. This man's association and support might act as a compensation of her long standing unfulfilled desire to get more and more attention from her dad.

Suspicious Scheme

"They refer to me, I feel, Dr.",—the client of the present vignette reported.

Question might be raised whether this is really a suspicious scheme and if so, where it is identical to suspiciousness noted in the paranoids. The important distinctions from the paranoid are—duration, intensity and associated symptoms. In the paranoid type, persecutory delusions are present. The delusions are dominated by the themes of (Suinn, 1975; Kleinmuntz, 1970) grandiosity and persecution (an unsubstantiated fear that the client will be harmed or persecuted by others). Associated with this is the theme related hallucinations (auditory). Negative symptoms are not displayed.

One might think again whether the symptom reported by the above case tallies well with the classical bookcase of schizophrenia. And again, whether her's are totally somatic concerns? The duration of schizophrenia must be more than 6 months, whereas, somatoform disorders must exist substanitally at least for a month or even less, if successfully treated (Grey and Zide, 2008).

The client's statement 'the girls, I think, are referring to me', is given so much importance here, because as a learner one must be sure whether the client's use of the term 'refer', denotes delusion at all. If it is truly delusion, we cannot miss such a diagnosis even for a day; because it will be detrimental to the client if adequate care is not provided with. The present client neither required any pharmacological treatment before, nor had her complaint prevailed for a month in her. This was an idea in her; she presumed that her roommates knew about her parents' matter and started discussing about it. The source of such leakage of information she reported could be her office colleagues, because she has disclosed this information to her boss, as she was finding it difficult for her to continue office work for late hours due to difficulty in concentration and sleep disturbance (again dependency and support seeking behaviour expressed).

In some cases paranoid attitudes may be expressed which is due to previous personality traits (Hamilton, 1976). They are likely to misinterpret easily environmentally justified reactions also. But in such cases paranoid ideas are rarely well-help delusions (Hamilton, 1976) In some cases such misinterpretation is precipitated by the client's prevailing mood. In this connection the reader may be reminded of a syndrome called 'paranoid depression', by Kraepelin (1921). This is characterised by marked depression and paranoid ideas, but associated symptoms are—agitation, severe suicidal thoughts, and auditory hallucinations. The latter symptoms were not present in the case being discussed now; nor the intensity of depression reported in the case was 'severe' enough to lead to suicidal attempts.

Some patients with moderately severe to severe level of anxiety or depression show marked delusions of persecution (Hamilton, 1976), which are not considered justified by them. These patients, as reported by Hamilton (1976), protest bitterly about the persecution and frequently attribute their depressive symptoms to their disturbing nature. The case illustration given here, first of all, did not have any persecutory delusion. Secondly, her depression was not very severe. Thirdly, suicidal thoughts were not present in her. This may be an exaggeration of life-long personality traits. Hamilton (1976) described the personality characteristics of such patients as—sensitive, introverted, quiet, paranoid, and keeps their paranoid ideas to themselves. These ideas become pronounced under the influence of events which cause anxiety and depression in them. It is possible, as Hamilton (1976) stated, that anxiety itself may play a part both in causing and exacerbation of ideas of reference. Hamilton (1976) also stated that such ideas of reference "because of its effect on goal-directed thinking, may prevent from thinking out the inaccuracy of her beliefs" (p. 96).

For the case under reference, it was not ideas of reference in actuality. The source of disclosure of personal information was the client herself. This was an apprehension; such inaccuracy in thinking the client has been able to identify herself and could rectify in the subsequent sessions of counselling. She did not require any pharmacological aid for amelioration of her complaints. Furthermore, the present case under reference appears to have such a feeling because of her passive aggressive personality trait. The paranoid personality in true sense accepts premises that others are hostile towards him and would take advantage of him. This, in other words, is a reflection of the more severe disturbance in him, known as 'paranoid psychotic state' (Suinn, 1975). In the latter, corresponding personality traits are displayed. Some such characteristics are—suspiciousness, distrustful, hypersensitive, tends to ascribe evil motives to others, envious and jealous of better treatments they think others receive, so he prefers to discontinue interaction with others. In the present case the above-mentioned traits were not present. The client, on the contrary showed a need to have interaction with others, and felt deserted when her roommates left her alone (reason not known to the client). But the same roommates used to talk to her when they used to come across with each other in office situations. May be the client's nature to refrain from discussions related to the persons of the opposite sex made her roommates feel awkward to discuss such matters with her. The passive-aggressive personality, under similar situations, may be compelled to leave a particular association but feels hurt if excluded, still the person is found to be interested in retaining contact with others, whilst the paranoid personality may eventually find all such encounters very unsatisfactory (Suinn, 1975)—may be because the client feels threatened. Secondly, the paranoid personality appears to suffer more in his interaction with others, the passive-aggressive personality seems to create more discomfort amongst those

(Suinn, 1975) who he thinks frustrate him. The case in illustration had not reported delusions of grandeur.

Such provisional categorisation helps the clinician to avoid arriving at a premature conclusion about a person's behaviour.

Synthesis

Here is a young lady with—(i) feeling of inferiority; (ii)) helplessness; (iii) sense of rejection due to absence of adequate attention, and (iv) strong resistance.

Resistance means that the client accepts distress at the conscious level, but denies to relate its content with the 'self' (defence?). Why defend? This has a psychosocial bearing. The client has a need to be socially associated and morally correct. It may be confusing to a learner that when a client has such a need why does the client feel rejected? Rejection is just an expression of a need for security.

Inferiority indicates helplessness to her relative smallness. Now question comes : What is her personality about? Is it dependent personality? Central characteristics of dependent personality are (i) difficulty in making decision; (ii) excessive need for reassurance; (iii) fear of rejection and abandonment; (iv) Not uncommon for such individuals to live with someone who is controlling, domineering, overprotective. These characteristics have been discussed in detail in the section devoted to differential assessment.

T = (i) **Termination**—Has to be intimated to the client well before the end. Sudden termination is not desired.

(ii) **Time**—Duration of each session and number of sessions to be covered (no commitment about the approximate number of sessions be given). Bridging the past and future via present—be done through the sessions. This is the whole idea behind conducting counselling sessions.

I = **Insight**—by the time elapsed, the client is supposed to have developed insight into his/her problems. Number of sessions, accordingly time taken to develop insight, might vary depending upon the strategy involved in the counselling procedure.

N = **New Life.** Such an experience by the client is an indication that the counselling sessions have come to an end successfully and the client has attained NEW LIFE by gaining insight.

G = **Goal.** This is the whole aim of conducting such sessions—that the client has been able to reach the desired goal and the counsellor has been successful in assessing the client to end his/her pursuit fruitfully.

Chapter 13

PHASES IN COUNSELLING

As face is the index of mind, an individual's behaviour is an index of his attitude towards oneself. An individual who has respect for himself can show respect to others. Therefore, to have change in a given individual's behaviour (attitude) toward others we need to help that individual change his own attitude towards himself/herself.

Normally, an individual's behaviour is supposed to be consistent with his self-concept. Need gratification, which is the nucleus of human life, has to be consistent with one's self-concept. Therefore, the self strives for consistency. Inconsistency, i.e., lack of congruence between experience and the self-concept, leads to maladjustment.

Conflict arises when introjected values are not in agreement with the true values. An individual in such cases reports that he doesn't know what he really wants. A self which has a sound structure doesn't experience any distortion. Of course, in day to day life new experiences are encountered. They are perceived to bear some relationship to the self. If no relationship with the self is perceived, those are ignored. Such experiences are thus denied, as those are perceived inconsistent with the self-structure. Thus, desirable changes in behaviour, can be brought through counselling—by altering the concept of the self. Altering the self-concept is really a very hard task and requires time. However, counselling process has to pas through certain stages.

Initial Phase

Stage 1 : Though the counsellor knows that the counselee is in a state of incongruence, usually, the counselee doesn't perceive such incongruence. As a result, many a times the clients do not recognise the need for counselling and do not volunteer for such help. The counsellor must be ready to accept such an unagreeable atmosphere at this stage.

The client's personal constructs are found to be extremely rigid. Such rigidity causes blockage in internal communication (reviewing of the subjective world) on the one hand, and, on the other, to induce a desire to change the experiential field in connection with the others.

Since the client doesn't recognise any problem, close and communicative relationship are often viewed as dangerous by the client. They are unwilling to communicate about personal matters : communication, if any, at all is only about external, impersonal matters, which have no apparent significance to the counsellor.

The counsellor must not be disappointed; must not perceive such an atmosphere as a failure, and must not also attribute this to his ownself (as limitation of the self). More the resistance on the part of the client to communicate, the higher should be the intuition of the counsellor to find ways to make the counselee communicative. An experienced counsellor can indeed help the client to break such resistance so much so that the client would succumb to the counsellor unveiling all his internal world.

For example, a 26 yr male, scientist with bright career, employed in a corporate organisation, unmarried, came for consultation with the complaints that he is being deprived by his office with regard to his placement whereas his colleagues with inferior quality have got better placement. He started feeling very insulted and got involved in altercation with his office boss. During interview he was found to be highly defensive, and used to deny throughout that he has any fault in being deprived of such opportunities. But interview revealed that he has had feelings of inferiority, suspiciousness (evident from contradictory statements), and body language indicated high internal arousal due to suppressed aggression, though he completely denied all these. He reported that his sleep is disturbed. This was used as a cue by the counsellor and the session continued with a discussion on the possible reasons for sleep disturbance in general (not referring to the client). While discussing, after sometime, the client hinted upon that he had problems with his parents; on enquiry he stated "Doctor, it is a value clash". He blamed both his parents, and expressed the need to bring the parents for consultation. The counsellor agreed upon a discussion with his parents. The client did it with a view to prove that he has not got any personal problem, rather it is his parents who require consultation. This, however, shows that the client had been emotionally aroused and wants to discuss certain things with the counsellor though apparently he may resist to take up his personal matters for discussion. Thus, the initial stage ends with a tone of success that the counsellor has been able to make the client prepared mentally to come for discussion in subsequent sessions.

For the counsellor, as a precaution, it seems better to remain non-committal in certain aspects of the client's views, in the initial phase. For example, when the client stated that his parents require consultation, in reply, instead of giving him a definite direction to bring the parents in the next session itself, he was told, "OK, if you so desire, you may bring them in the subsequent sessions". This was so stated because the counsellor could understand that as long as the client shifts blames onto others, its implicit meaning is that the client has realised (but wants to forget/suppressed) that he too has some fault in causing his present distress. If the counsellor emphasises more to bring his parents in the next session itself, that will develop further resistance in the client to attend the session subsequently. The client is apprehensive that what all he wants to suppress now will be revealed through his parents to the counsellor.

In sum, it is the task of the counsellor in the initial session to see that he/she can motivate the client to continue subsequent sessions of counselling, no matter whether the client wants to discuss personal or impersonal matters. It is, again, the task of the counsellor to help the counselee to open up for discussing personal matters later, though initial discussion of impersonal matters may be of some help in this pursuit.

Stage 2 : Assumptions prior to the session : Prior to the initiation of the session, it is advisable on the part of the counsellor to assume—(i) whether the outcome of the ensuing session would be successful, (ii) what the counsellor expects the counselee's reaction would be in this session as aftermath of the initial session, (iii) which are the areas the counsellor requires to focus upon in this session, and (iv) how far the client will cooperate.

In continuance of Stage 1, it was expected that the counselee would begin to speak about matters which are remote in relation to his ownself. He won't bring his parents, will be further defensive in revealing the truth.

As expected, to start with, the counselee raised some questions on the issues discussed in the initial stage. Such a query, once again, in an indication, that the counselee has started thinking within himself about the genesis of his personal problems based on the previous discussion (initial stage) though still showing resistance to open up full. Secondly, he appeared to be very rigid in holding his personal views unchanged, and showed avoidance in taking any responsibility on himself in connection with his problems (i.e., a tendency to blame others was apparent once again). Thirdly, the client—though expressed his desire to bring his parents for counselling in the next session, as expected—did not bring them. On enquiry stated that "Doctor, on second thought I decided to bring them later." This shows that—(i) the client fails to keep up his commitment (purposive behaviour?); (ii) he might have thought that during interview with his parents some of his personal problems might come to the limelight (tendency to conceal fact); (iii) following his rigid constructs, he is again taking him away from a free expression of his main problem (avoidance of self-blame).

Counselling for the client, in real sense of the term, cannot start at this stage also. But for that the counsellor need not be demotivated as because, the more the controversial issues the client brings for discussion, the more it indicates that the client is vacillating between either accepting or denying his problems fully. In fact, the client has started feeling within that he cannot totally deny that some sort of problems does exist in him (counsellor's assumption), though side-tracking the main issue in counselling session to avoid self-blaming.

In sum : Stage 2 ends with a 2-way gain—(a) the counselee is in a fix—whether to start discussing personal issues with the counsellor; (b) the counsellor gets more stronger excuses in his/her hand that he.she will be able to help the client to express his personal problems to the counsellor soon. Because, making delay on the part of the client is helpful in the sense that it prepares the client to surrender to the consultant for help shortly.

Stage 3 : Assumptions prior to the session : The client will countinue session; may be relatively little free to discuss; lots of contradiction in thoughts may be revealed.

The client came on time and was found eager to sit for the session. To start with this session the client appeared to be relatively more free to continue discussion. Not only free, but a sense of submissiveness also was noticed in him. Submissiveness (though not the target of the counsellor to prove that the client submits to hjim thinking that the counsellor is superior) is likely to indicate helplessness in the client; that is, over the last two stages what all have been discussd those have given a sort of unsettling feeling in the client where he has started thinking that his rigid constructs may not be appreciated and accepted by others with whom he interacts in daily life.

It was discussd whethr as a result of his rigidity there may be any chances of his being victimised (e.g., in employment situation the authority may not comply with his rigid construct, consequently he might lose job).

At this juncture, some incongruence was evident in his thought and body language also. The client startednarrating how altercations took place between him and his boss. Thereafter he expressed that "Doctor, I'm not to create problem; better I will comply with the authority in occupational set-up; can you help me, doctor, to reinstate my position here?" At the next moment he said, "You know, doctor, for me it's no problem at all to get a job like that of the present status." The former statement expressed very well his feeling of helplesseness and tendency to succumb to the authority whilst the latter statement gave an impressjon that to succumb means to him a sense of failure, it is perceived as a loss by him. The client is in a fix now between feelings of helplessness versus non-acceptance of other support (support seeking = failure).

By this time it is clear to the counsellor that, out of basic inferiority and inadequacy feelings, the client has got the present problem. It is a clash with authority figure (not necessarily with his office boss, but quite likely with his parents and similar others as well), that is the reason that the client in the beginning stated that his parents require consultation.

In sum, this stage ends with a contradiction. Such an experience of contradiction in the counselee helps the counsellor to overcome his/her ambiguities, if any at all, and he/she can be sure that the counselee is half-way through to understand the content of discussion in the counselling sessions so far conducted. More the bifurcation in the client's behaviour, the more linear would be the counsellor's strategy for continuing the subsequent sessions.

Stage 4 : Assumptions prior to the session : (i) The client would be behaviourally relaxed and motivated to come for the session; (ii) the client will show resistance to accept self-blaming; (iii) to justify the present complaints; some association with the past life events would be required. But the counsellor in this regard remains in a dubious state, because the client may or may not cooperate. If the latter becomes true, then it would be clear to the counsellor that the client is apprehensive that his own fault may get revealed while narrating some of the significant and related past events in life. His non-cooperation would indicates his avoidance. May be administration of psychological test would be required. If the former is true, i.e., the client understands the relevance of some such past life events in context to his present problems and wants to discuss, then the counsellor can assure himself/herself that the counselling process is almost half-way through, in the sense that the counselee has prepared himself to accept whatever comes out from such disclosure of his life events; thereby the counselee, unknowingly, helps the counsellor to enrich himself/herself with matters relevant for discussion in subsequent session.

Contrary to the pre-session assumptions, during the session, the above mentioned client was found late to report, and behaviourally was tensed : (A) that he was late to attend the session had significant implications to the counsellor—(i) the client is indecisive whether to continue counselling (conflict?); (ii) to kill the time scheduled for him, so that discussion of some intrinsic won't be possible (avoidance?).

(B) That he looked tensed, in spite of his relaxing attitude noted in the last session, would imply that—the discussion held in the last session has really stirred him up cognitively about the obscure matters behind his present problem which he doesn't want to bring to the surface (resistance?).

The counsellor must not be disappointed; rather should assure himself/herself that such conflict, avoidance, the resistance of the client can be dealt with in future sessions. The client, unknowingly, had agreed with the counsellor about the areas which require further probing, and the counsellor be thankful to the client for providing him/her with such valuable indications at an early phase of the counselling process.

To divert the attention of the counsellor the client raised an altogether separate issue in his session. That is, "Doctor, should I resign from my service?" Counsellor—"Let us see what prompted you to think so". What are the possible reasons for his having such an impulsive thought were discussed; enquiry was done again on his office related matters and matters related to his home front.

The trend of the discussion was to relate the life incidents together, instead of taking each event, namely, office or home related events as discrete phenomenon. The client reciprocated well during the time left for this session, and looked much less tensed at the end of the session. He fixed up next appoint himself.

Stage 5 : Assumptions prior to the session : (i) The client will be motivated to come for the session; (ii) will cooperate to discuss obscure events of life.

The case under reference was found waiting outside the counsellor's office prior to the latter's arrival (could it be eagerness on the part of the client?). The client was found relaxed and cooperative. Discussion was held on his family structure and environment in detail. He started blaming his father, and his mother and also both of their family members. It could be revealed that, as he feels, both of his patents have failed to take right decisions many a times about him. Also, to him, both the parents are biased to some extent in providing priority to other family members (where the client has had experienced neglected), and thus he has lost his trust on them. He had a feeling since childhood that his mother is more reasonable compared to his father but of late has started thinking that his mother too is equally unreasonable (narrated some incidents to justify such comments) like his father, and, as such, he has lost confidence in the parents; he has developed aggression towards them.

The three most important implications of the above are—(i) the client has a tendency to blame others (if at all the incidents/events he narrated are true; thus it requires verification and confirmation from the parents); such a tendency helps him to rationalise his present problems. He seems to say that his present problem is nothing but an offshoot of his parental interaction pattern with him since childhood.

(ii) The client has recognised the root of his problems associating the past and the present, but doesn't want to confess it directly even now.

(iii) The client has lost trust in his parents (probably because he has lost trust in himself).

The counsellor's gain—he could help the client associate the past and the present (no incident/event he perceived as a discrete phenomenon in life, as discussed in the previous phase).

The client's gain—even if his parents are responsible for his present problem, just to blame them would not help him in any way. The client has to understand how he can solve his present problem and can enrich his self-esteem.

In sum : This phase is devoted to help the client understand : (i) some of his rigid personal constructs in relation to his interaction pattern with others; (ii) can understand contradictions in personal choices in a better way; (iii) can prepare himself to find the weaknesses of his personal decision making power in its proper perspective. Despite this the client may somehow perceive the self (—adopted to (i), (ii) and (iii)—as an object (the counsellor's realisation), which is separate from his actual self.

Middle Phase

Stage 6 : Assumptions prior to the session : (i) The client's tendency to shift blame to others can be realised by him; (ii) The client can realise and accept his own contributions to his present problem(s); (iii) Under what circumstances an individual perceive self as an object—be the main theme of discussion.

The counsellor begins this session with an idea in mind that the client's perception of the self must be subjective. An expert professional can make the client understand incongruence between the client's experiences and the client's perception of the self. The client can express his experiences of the present and becomes gradually less bound by the past structure of blaming others. The client can overcome his defences, at least occasionally, in this session. But still distrust prevails; which leads to fear of humiliation. The client learns to take self-responsibility for his problems but vacillates over the sessions, and during the session also.

For example, the above case expressed the following contradictions in this session :

(i) He has a very high drive for academic and professional achievements (for social reputation), but at the same time he feels that people (particularly authority figure) may not have confidence into him (inferiority?); (ii) he thinks he can achieve what he wants to, but lacks patience to keep pace with the time; (iii) the client said, "I feel I must follow what the authority wants me to do (social desirability), but sometimes I feel they humiliate me (inferiority leading to suspiciousness?)", because information received from his office doesn't show any resonance with the client's stated views (as the counsellor feels); (iv) "I will expose the authority" (need to proof superiority/power?); "doesn't matter even if I've to resign" (need to prove his authenticity); at the same session expressed that it was his dream to work in an organisation like the one he is attached with now.

In sum : In such cases information from different sources must be gathered prior to blaming the client as suspicious, inferior etc. However, discussion on such issues helps the client develop better understanding and to move in the direction of professional counselling to ameliorate the problem. Still the client may appear to be cautious in establishing a therapeutic relationship (lack of empathy? or due to suspiciousness?). Mention be made here that in Indian set-up, due to social stigma it is difficult normally to have an easy access to interact with the client's employer/colleagues, unless otherwise indicated. If, for example, an emotional outburst occurs in the office set-up itself, or else neither the patients/clients nor the guardians of them would like to ventilate such matters to the employers out of apprehension. It doesn't mean that the employers will not cooperate with the client. Mostly the employers provide all sorts of support to the client; but due to apprehension clients normally refrain from seeking such help. Disclosure of such information that the counsellor has consulted the employer/colleagues make the clients and their family more perturbed. With consent from the clients and their family members such intervention is advisable. For the case under reference information was gathered from the respective office of the client and his parents too. The employer did not reveal that negative an attitude towards the client that the client would be sacked (the client was apprehensive about it). In fact, the client was later offered onsite opportunities which indicates the mistrust noticed in the client was self-made. To avoid social humiliation the client even thought of submitting voluntarily resignation from the service.

Stage 7 : Assumptions prior to the session : (i) Residual resistance, if any, noticed in the client to reveal information—that has to be dealt with adequately; (ii) expected that the client will provide some more relevant information particularly concerning his pre-morbid characteristics.

By this time the counsellor must have clear idea about the hesitation of the client in becoming free while establishing a professional relationship in terms of verbal give and take. He has to deal with the residual resistance of the client which causes hindrance to be free. This shows that the client thus can't accept all his feelings as his own, still distrust, contradictions, and lack of clarity are present in him.

For example, the given case reported after so many sessions that he has inferiority, particularly with regard to his physical stature. He also expressed that such a feeling has been ingrained in him since his school days. The counsellor to discuss here whether the client's striving for achievement, social recognition, and impatience for better placement could be to compensate his inner feelings of inferiority (though he has achieved academically and vocationally more than the average). Also, the counsellor, at this juncture, should keep in mind whether such inferiority feeling with regard to one's physical stature could have any negative impact onto the client's role playing, particularly sex-role identity, and sex-role playing. The latter, if present, might give rise to suspiciousness in the client. In fact, the latter aspect turned out to be true in this case after the end of this session.

In sum : Though the client wants to express his/her feelings freely, some fear and distrust still prevail at the initial phase of this stage. Gradually, the client can accept incongruence in his experience; can learn to accept that his feelings are self-made (ingranied). He can accept events in life with responsibility. Thus, notable feature in this session is improvement in reducing blockage of internal communication, which paves way to establish a better professional relationship through free dialogue.

Stage 8 : Assumptions prior to the session : (i) Inhibitionfree communication would be possible; (ii) this would help understanding the client's personal orientation towards himself/herself and, consequently, facilitate his relationship with others; (iii) would consent to separate sessions with the parents.

The client is prepared now to express his feelings explicitly. He/she has been able to overcome inhibitions in communicating his/her feelings. The client also has made up his/her mind to express feelings immediately without any procrastination. This shows that the client is ready to accept thoughts/feelings as they occur, without any bias.

For e.g., the above cited case started discussing 'Do you know, doctor, now-a-days we get so much of information about everything through internet. It help us to enrich our knowledge quickly.' The counsellor—'Yes, I know'.

Counsellor—'Do you mean to discuss any specific issue in this context?'

Client—'Yes. You know, doctor, we get so many information about bisexuality, homosexuality (gay) etc. These things make me so much confused, you know, particularly in context to our culture. You know, I must go abroad, where I presume they don't bother about one's personal matters like gay or lesbian etc.

Counsellor—'Let's discuss what are the problems you face in Indian culture regarding the issue of sexuality/sexual orientation you have brought forward'.

From the above two very important points are worth mentioning :

(i) The client is totally free from hesitation and wants to discuss even core personal matters freely and immediately;

(ii) He has problems with regard to sexual orientation.

The client initially came with the complaints—feeling of being oppressed by the authority (in occupational sphere), feeling of rejection (his cognitive potentialities not acknowledged properly by the colleagues) and feeling of internal irritation leading to recent sleep disturbance. These complaints, though, appear to be apparently unrelated with the inner feelings he has expressed up to Stage 6, dynamically, those are meaningful to a counsellor. The counsellor has already realised that the roots of such complaints must lie somewhere in the client's personal life interaction process; particularly important here is the developmental phase of the counselee when his self-concept was developed. Since childhood he has been oppressed by his parents (as he stated before); that apprehension of oppression in exercising his individuality has been reflected onto his office boss and senior colleagues too. Also, his feeling of self-esteem and that of competency in role playing are inadequate. Thus, though apparently authority figure in occupational sphere, seems to have done injustice to him, actually it is the personal orientation of the client and his self-perception (inferiority) which illuminates and contaminates his perception of others' interaction towards him. When asked the client consented to call his parents but hesitantly.

In sum : Need for restructuring of the personal orientation of the client has been understood by the client himself.

End Phase

Stage 9 : Assumptions prior to session : (i) Communication would be fruitful to the extent that incongruence becomes congruence; (ii) would pave the way for the development of self-trust.

The client is in a position now to accept—and not to deny—contradictions noticed so far in his thoughts, feelings, and actions. He/she is no longer defensive to reveal negatives. Rather he/she is ready to accept negatives and to make them positive and hopeful. He/she prepares now onwards to take firm decisions and not to vacillate. He/she feels free to discuss and to find remedies for the problems experienced even now.

For example, in the above case, he accepted at this stage that he has had conflict with regard to his sexual orientation; narrated freely that he was afraid of his father since childhood and was relatively more close to his mother but experienced a sort of alienation in the family. Never he was allowed to interact with girls; had homosexual experiences in school-days. Later he tried heterosexual relations with same-age girls and with elderly women but always experienced failure; with the same-age people this was out of fear of humiliation that they may approach him but he is not knowledgeable as to how to reciprocate. He was relatively relaxed with elderly females but in none of the cases he was satisfied. With the elderly he experienced very delayed ejaculation occasionally, but mostly no ejaculation. He fantasised that young boys of his age would be a better and easy partner for him, though occasionally experienced his feeling to be heterosexual (to conform to social norm). Discussion continued to decide upon his future orientation in this regard; accordingly he could be helped.

In sum : The client was prepared to accept his liabilities and assets as they are. He agreed that the counsellor could talk to his parents also.

Stage 10 : Assumptions prior to session : (i) Would provide consent to guide him to decide upon his future orientation, particularly in relation to sex; (ii) would accept the need to be assertive but not aggressive as and when necessary; (iii) reorientation of self-esteem would be possible.

Due to widening of the cognitive maps of his self-experience, the feelings are now accepted and owned. Due to breaking of rigid boundaries the client experiences change in the manner of his interaction with others. There is a change in his manner and style of attributing meaning to the inputs he/she receives through interaction with others. The client is ready to accept himself/herself as subject and not as an object.

For example, in the above-cited case—the client experience that he has understood that he must not go for any confrontation with the authority in the office (place of his occupation). If he wants to fulfil his desires, better to get it done through understanding his colleagues rather than challenging. He realised that he might have interpreted other's way of dealing with him in a biased way. The client said, "Let me prove my efficiency better, to impress them (authority) and thus to get my desire fulfilled through them". Counselling also helped him to understand the reasons for his developing ambivalent attitude towards selection of partner in sexual interaction. He expressed the desire to refrain from homosexual relationship and to provide sufficient positive thoughts to his sex related imagination about his competency and adequacy.

In sum : Self-realisation is a focal theme here. Self as an object thus tends to disappear.

Stage 11 : Assumptions prior to session : (i) Would reciprocate well during discussion session; (ii) would show conviction to trust himself.

Since the client has been able to assess, by now, his/her assets and liabilities both, and also that he/she has realised limitations of his/her on in interpreting life events and executing the same in real life situations, it makes the client ready to revisit his/her cognitive map, and, when necessary, to re-draw it to get it matched with the demands of reality. That is, the client has been able to develop trust onto himself/herself, which, in turn, will help him/her not to mistrust others without sufficient and genuine reasons. Counselling thus helps developing respect for one's own self as well as for the self of others.

For example, the above cited case now started interaction with colleagues without aggressing them. Likewise, in the family front also, a shift in his attitude was observed. Earlier, the client, though had himself suggested the need for joint sessions with parents (the request was superficial), had avoided them out of the fear that his hidden wishes will be resolved in front of them (conflict). Now, he not only agreed for (conflict resolution), but even fixed up a date for joint sessions (took an initiative). The client is now found free from initial resistance he had shown to initiate discussion in counselling sessions; he has shown interest to take up certain issues on his on for discussion. The client also has shown interest to report for follow-up session for sometimes more. Pre-sessional assumptions were fulfilled.

In sum : Self-actualisation by the client is the main focus here.

Stage 12 : Assumptions prior to session : (i) Joint session with the parents would be fruitful; (ii) if necessary parents may be interviewed separately, for which the client is expected to consent without any hesitation.

The client came on time along with his parents. The client consented for taking separate sessions also with the parents, if the counsellor deems it suitable (trusts on to the counsellor developed). After a brief session with the client, the parents were advised about certain lapses and gaps, the client expressed in their interactional process since his childhood. The parents accepted it. The parents were called for separate sessions individually. Then the joint session with the parents taken. Occasionally, between parents, contradictions arose in deciding over some of the issues—those were dealt with accordingly. The session was windedup taking a joint session of the parents and the client together—so that they can help each other to reinstate the happiness and mental strength of the client and also of the parents. They were advised to continue follow up sessions.

Follow-up sessions

To start with, separate session with each of the parents (if necessary), be taken, or joint session with the parents separately and with the client separately be taken. Later sessions, in follow-up, be taken together. Six months to 1 yr intermittent follow-up is advised for relapse prevention.

After the first follow-up session the client got placed abroad on the same service and thus subsequent sessions with him had not been possible. Parents used to meet the counsellor meticulously during follow-up and used to inform about the client's quality of life in abroad. As stated by the parents, both of them and also their son are happy now.

In sum : There is no specific phase or any specific stage either which is strategic for counselling. In any counselling it is conventional to think of the phases and/or stages depending upon the strategy to the emoluments. Generally, phases may broadly be divided into—initial, mid, and end phase. The whole strategy depends largely upon the nature of the client, the degree of the client's problems and the specialisation of the counsellor in selecting the technique to be employed. The present chapter provides some hints to the trainees as to how to proceed for reconciliation after estrangement—particularly for the clients having multiple problems and that too in different spheres of their life.

Chapter 14

GROUP COUNSELLING

Group counselling may be considered as an extension of individual counselling. In such a set-up free communication between members (if required, 2 or more members) and amongst members (entire group) is felt essential and encouraged. Such free communication helps understanding each other's problems and thereby facilities understanding of one's own problems quickly and in a better way. Heated emotions get cooled off soon which paves way for discussion. Discussion helps understanding each one's role in creating one's own problems as well as in the amelioration of the problems.

Groups may differ from one another in many respects, namely, primary group, secondary group, and out-group. Primary group ordinarily comprises of members of a family, though not necessarily always. Structural arrangement of the group and characteristics of the members who constitute the group are of main concern in it; this is more so in respect to group therapy. Be it group therapy or counselling, group must be small in size and constituents of the group should have similar problems. Participants must be homogeneous with respect to their problems, age, education, intelligence, language, etc. In family counselling of a particular family, or in counselling for children's problems the group is heterogeneous in respect of age, sex, and education of the members. However, group counselling cannot be resorted to for any and every kind of problem.

Indian Scenario

In general, people show lot of resistance of receive counselling individually. More resistance is expressed ordinarily by the clients to sit in a group for such assistance, particularly in non-institutional set-up. This is because there used to prevail a misconception that receiving counselling means the counselee be labelled as 'abnormal'. However, in recent years, the term counselling has been popular with regard to career counselling and youths are relatively more free to come for such kind of assistance. Sometimes our younger generation, though, intend to come for clinical counselling, initially portray a totally different picture. That is, they come with a plea of vocational, or career counselling, etc. and gradually express their deep-rooted personal conflicts. In some cases where a couple agrees to come for counselling together, for e.g., marital counselling, that in itself forms a group. Otherwise, for adolescents and young adults, family counselling (in a group) sometimes is possible to arrange for, only after receiving consent from the other members. Mostly consent seeking takes longtime, particularly for adolescence and young adults. Such resistance is mainly because of lack of trust. Clients are afraid that their private and confidential matters may divulge easily through such group discussion. However, integration group sessions with individual counselling session are found effective in many cases. But group counselling is contraindicated for individuals with serious psychological problems (Rao, 1981), particularly for the persons with deep unconscious conflicts. In no case should group counselling be considered a substitute for individual counselling. In practice, however, both the methods are used to supplement each other, provided the counsellor's expertise deems it suitable.

Group therapy is helpful in many instances. For example, multiple family counselling in which a number of families are brought together from simultaneous counselling. But in Indian set-up, family members show lot of resistance for such open discussions. This is not much in vogue compared to single family meeting for counselling. As mentioned before, there too, adolescence and young adults show strong resistance to sit for open discussion with their parents and family members. It is a time-consuming process for the counsellor to prepare such clients for family counselling together. In hospital set-up, particularly in family wards, arrangement is made sometimes for group discussion with members of different families and their parents together. However, that becomes more of a group therapy rather than counselling. Discussion of group therapy is beyond the scope of the book.

In clinical counselling with individual clients it is often evident that there is much more to be unveiled beyond what the client had expressed as problem. Most problem behaviours are products of problem homes. Disturbed home environment affects the harmonious development of the individual. Problem behaviour, thus, is a symptom of a sick system. In this sense, each client reflects a family. Parent(s) counselling deals with the areas of sibling rivalry, parent-child relationship concerning the dimension of dependence-independence, autonomy-submission, and regarding conflicts concerning vocational choice, life achievement, marriage, and so on. Mostly, nowadays, parents become unrealistic in their demands on their offsprings with regard to educational and vocational choices which causes frustration in the clients as well as in their parents. Quite often parents try to compensate their personal life failures through the achievements of their children which causes several problems to the children when they grow-up. That is why family counsel' ıg for each client becomes a part of the whole counselling process. Unfortunately this area has received minimal attention as because, in Indian society, particularly in industrial areas, it becomes difficult to get all the members of a family together. Secondly, many a times, members of a family are found reluctant to sit together for counselling with the apprehension of getting family secrecy unveiled. Thus, we need to organise more and more public awareness programmes to make people motivated to understand the utility of counselling which in turn will motivate them to come forward for consultation. One cannot, in counselling, really compartmentalise an individual (the client), and his family as separate systems and his/her culture as the third system. Much work has to be done with cultural factors in counselling. Thus, an ecological perspective in family counselling has to be emerged, an issue which was raised by Ackerman long ago (1970).

Marriage Counselling

This is another set-up where the situation itself demands joint counselling sessions—at least for 2 individuals together (if not more, when family members are also to be included). Many a times, when a couple comes for counselling together, it is found that they don't fulfil the inclusion criteria necessary for enrolment to marital counselling programme. Some such criteria are dissimilarities in attitude and interests for the partners causing interactional difficulties, when one of the spouses is with high level of anxiety, depression, suspiciousness and OCD like problems; or any physical illness, the course, management and prognosis of which is not known to the other partner, and the like. Counselling is required for infertility related stress, and for enrichment of knowledge regarding availability and implementation of modern technology in its treatment and also regarding its side-effects.

There are, of course, certain contraindications for marital counselling. **From the couple's point of view**—when one of the partners is either unwilling or unable to participate in the sessions. When one of the partners reveals discomfort in anticipation that the counsellor will favour the partner of the same sex in solving problems of the couple. Intense negative counter-transference (Karpel, 1994) is also contraindicative.

From the counsellor's point of view—It is advisable not to accept the couple for such services with whom the counsellor has either had any previous alliance or breach of ethics (Cameron, Ennis and Deadman, 1998). Likewise, it is advisable not to establish such professional relationship with relatives, friends, office-colleagues, and others well-known to the counsellor, on ethical ground.

It once again requires expertise on the part of the clinical counsellor to realise and also to make the couple understand that it is not the relationship (as marriage) which requires counselling, but individual characteristics of each of the partners of a couple require counselling. The counsellor has to make it clear to the couple that had they been married to some other persons, there to, problems would have been evident in their adjustment, unless the couple change some of their basic personality qualities. The counsellor's objective is to reform them and not to make them conform. In many instances, marriage counselling turns out to be individual-counselling. The counsellor has to exercise his skills with utmost care and, perhaps, client-centred approach is most appropriate in this regard, provided the clients are matured from academic point of view to realise the cause-and-effect relationship of their problems. Otherwise non-directive approach is employed. After a few sessions of individual counselling, couple could be ready to sit for marital counselling jointly.

Marriage counselling has three important areas, namely, (i) premarital counselling, (ii) counselling for a better marital adjustment, (iii) counselling to save a marriage from breaking down.

(i) **Premarital Counselling :** This is a very vital stage in determining whether marriage will be successful. The counsellor helps the would be partners to gain a complete understanding of themselves; this is in terms of their compatibilities and incompatibilities with regard to their basic needs and demands in life, philosophy of life, and nature of personality as a whole. Affairs, which are totally based on physical attraction and/or biological need gratification, cannot last long. What is essential in sustaining a marriage peacefully is empathetic understanding towards each other. This is necessary because in India live-together system is not much in vogue with the exception of a few cases where situation has become very rare. Such understanding can develop only when the partners can follow the given sequence during their courtship stage.

Not to be overwhelmed by physical attractiveness, materialistic comforts like financial assets, and reputation of the person. These help in forming fanciful and myopic understanding only, which is superficial. One must remember that empathy is in no way parallel to superficial beauty. Real beauty is always skindeep.

They must look for exploring compatibility in value system of each other. This is possible only when one becomes concerned to explore fundamental incompatibilities between them. When incompatibilities are uncovered, depending upon its nature and extent one has to decide whether in future they can really exchange their views in the pursuit of having reliable emotional support for each other, sharing responsibilities and executing adequate role playing in their life. Compatibility in values be checked through attitudes towards life achievements, gender role, financial status, sex role, family planning, leisure activities, religion, politics, age, socialisation and so forth.

Premarital counselling and Indian scenario

Unlike the Western societies, the Indian social customs don't allow a period of courtship. Though the situation is changing now-a-days, even then, in the Indian society most marriages are arranged, and partners, more often than not, are complete strangers to each other. In this sense future of the partners is left absolutely on chance factor as to whether the relationship will be a happy one. Contrary to the expectation, relatively more rate of divorce is recorded with couples having love marriage compared to those of arranged marriage. This shows that the so-called love is at the superficial level. Our adolescents and young adults fail to understand each other in real sense. They become convinced by some fanciful misconceptions, bodily attractions, etc. Many a times, without the consent of their parents, such partners go for marriages, but within a short while marriage turns out to be a failure. This is because young partners being involved emotionally, cannot judge adequately the family background, family upbringing process, attitude of family members toward the daughter-in-law/son-in-law, attitude towards each other on psychological perspective, and many such other issues necessary for leading a happy marital life. Moreover, even now, most of the families in India have a desire to live in a joint family system, if not the son is employed in a different place outside his home town/village. Many a times, it is reported that out of a pressure created by the daughter-in-law the married son starts living separately with his wife (leaving his parents), but it creates guilt in the son that he is doing injustice to his parents; and, as such, gradually misunderstanding develops between the couple. Such attitudinal differences between the partners are to be clarified in premarital counselling so that the marriage does not end abruptly. But very rarely would the couples come for premarital counselling in Indian set-up. Because, many of them are not aware of the availability of such services, and also the necessity of such services. Some of them think that coming for counselling could mean that they have problems, they are ill, and become apprehensive that affair may end abruptly if they consult a counsellor. Thirdly, since courtship is not yet accepted by many parents in India, the partners do not come for counselling thinking that parents will be able to know about their affair and it will break. Indian society has conventional and traditional views of—and attitude towards—marriage. Marriage is not considered merely as a matter concerning two individuals, but is looked upon as an event which involves families and communities at large. Thus, the question of individual choice of partner is limited. Though the situation is changing now, parents do have expectation that they will be involved directly in the selection of their son's/daughter's life partner and also that after marriage their son will live with them in a joint family set-up, if not otherwise warranted. Thus, consent and approval of the family and acceptance of the new member in the family becomes the desideratum.

Counselling for a better marital adjustment

Obviously premarital counselling provides a better opportunity to understanding each other well before the partners start family life, and, as such, there is wide scope for modification of each others' attitude such that mutual bonds of liking and affection can grow.

In marriage counselling, when partners complain of difficulties in adjustment, precipitating events be elicited first and dealt with accordingly. Because prevention be given first priority, intervention aspect can be dealt with later. Precipitating events would cover, on the one hand, individual factors from the point of view of each partner, and, on the other, environmental factors. Individual factors, namely, are—nature of employment of the husband and the wife and time they have to spend outside the family; if wife is employed, than husband's expectation from her in looking after the family, chronic illness in the family, illness of life partner and its prognosis; financial crisis in the family, if any; economic independence of the wife (particularly when the wife is unemployed; of course many a times it is reported that the wife, though employed, does not have economic independence because of the in-laws' encroachment in her personal matters); social freedom of the wife; level of aspiration whether fulfilled with regard to both the partners; sex conflict; sexual problems, attitude toward parenthood, gender discrimination with regard to offsprings, etc. Environmental factors—crisis in marriage arise in our society, mostly due to intrusion of a third party; e.g., in-laws, or unmarried sister in the husband's family; married sister with a tendency to control over the brotner's family unit; intrusion of relatives in the personal matters of the married couple etc. These can cause emotional turmoil leading to a crisis.

Personality predispositions of both the partners are also to be looked into. Marriage can sustain well—provided compatibilities are more in number between partners than incompatibilities. The partners should be similar in attitudes, interests, culture, value system and so on. They must lean on empathy with adequate communication between them. Age is another important factor for compatibility. Now-a-days lower age gap between life partners is preferred.

The counsellor helps the couple understand each other, their basic needs, drives and requirements. Each of the partners must be able to develop attitude that he/she seeks from the other. They must learn to be more logical and also be in a position to see that emotion does not overpower their decision-making process.

In short : The counsellor aims to help the partners unveil and realise the incompatibilities that prevail in them.

Of course, the counsellor must be very clear about his/her role and also to make it clear to the couple that the counsellor's task is not to provide them ready solutions to their problems. The counsellor is not an arbitrator. His/her role is not to tell what is right for them. His/her role is to help the partners understand each other—providing them a sense of orientation. Such an approach of the counsellor enables the couple to believe that a solution has to be found on the basis of their involvement to the relationship. Perhaps client-centred approach is most appropriate in this regard, provided the couple fulfil the inclusion criteria necessary for such approach.

Many a times the counsellor has to face problems with resistant clients. The counsellor must have mental preparation that the clients may not volunteer to provide him/her relevant information; the counsellor has to elicit it skilfully. Mostly people are found to have narrow vision. They fail to recognise and/or refuse to recognise their own faults and weaknesses. The counsellor has to help the couple discover himself/herself his/her shortcomings in maintaining marital relationship. Needless to mention that the clients will volunteer to provide information only when they will be sure about the professional expertise of the counsellor, and also the counsellor's approach in maintaining confidentiality and other ethical codes. In other words, when the clients can develop confidence on the counsellor in every respect, rapport in real sense of the term is established and thereby the client prepares himself/herself to reach the counsellor.

The counsellor in marital counselling may have to refer the couple to other specialists, namely, a physician, a sexologist, a psychiatrist or any such other speciality, if necessary, for verification and confirmation of such related problems in marital adjustment reported by the couples. In case of any gynaecological problem, the counsellor will have to advice the client to receive necessary treatment by the respective physicians but emotional problems arising out of such issues are to be dealt with adequate skill by the counsellor.

To save marriage from break-up

When couple has experienced prolonged furstration due to incompatibilities in their personality dispositions or due to socio-economic circumstances, or due to some such other matters, then the question of break-up arises. How to forestall a marriage from break-up? In such a situation marriage counselling is looked upon as a form of crisis intervention. In such cases, many a times couple complaints of associated psychiatric problems, viz., sleep disturbance, low mood, lack of energy in work etc. Accordingly, advice from a psychiatrist should be sought for to help the client ameliorate such secondary symptoms. It is possible, though very difficult and time taking, to forestall a marriage from break-up by helping the couple realise their deep level need to leave the given partner and to look for a second.

Case Illustration

(1) Woman—36, graduate, engaged in the progession of Fine Arts, got married (love marriage) 6 yrs earlier with a man (about 43 yrs) of her same profession. First conception was aborted with her consent and they do not have any issue till now. She is at present depressed and desperate to leave her husband. On inquiry it could be revealed (with lots of resistance) that she has developed inclination towards another man. Counselling was centred around whethr personality predisposition of the woman drives her to shift from one man to another. Such depth interpretation later helped her to continue meaningful life with the present husband.

(2) A software ennngineer, 28 yrs, got married-to-a postgraduate girl of 24. It is a negotiated marriage, both from well to do families. At present thety have a baby (son, $1^1/_2$ yrs) and duration of their marriage is 5 years. After marriage the wife got a job (teaching at the secondary level). On day one, they had experienced some misunderstanding between them and subsequent unhappiness. They complained of no financial crisis, or any such other problems which could jeopardise their relationship. In spite of having everything necessary to live a comfortable life, why were they not happy that was rather their main concern. Both the partners are very dutiful to others but fail to adequately perform duties to each other because of their inner aggression. The wife complained that her husband was indifferent to her, and the husband complained that the wife was immature.

On inquiry it was found that the husband has had very bright career, deeply engrossed in his own education and profession, prefers to have minimum interaction with others, reserved, shy, but stubborn. The wife, on the other hand, prefers more social interactions, happy-go-lucky type; even if misunderstanding occurs with her husband, after a short period of silence she takes initiative to mitigate it. But the husband never takes initiative in this regard even if he is at fault.

In short, marital disharmony was due to personality (ego) clash between the husband—who is an extreme introvert—and the wife—an extrovert.

Husband's indifferent attitude was found to be generalised and not particularly towards his wife only. During counselling, when this could be revealed, the wife could realise her misinterpretation that husband does not show any interest in her. The husband was also helped through counselling to realise that he has to modify his style of life in terms of sharing ideas and family duties with his wife, to spend time with his wife and son. Once again, apparent misunderstanding based on certain situational issues is due to deep-rooted personality problems of the couple.

(3) A man (31 yrs), married (spouse is 26) since lst 6 years; love marriage, having courtship period for a short duration, having two daughters; husband is a businessman and wife is a service holder; joint family. Gradually husband has started being indifferent towards his wife; conseuently wife has become easily irritable and aggressive.

Since the husband was found to be highly defensive during initial interview, and the wife was found to be totally shattered through husband's domination and misbehaviour, it seemed justified to administer psychological tests to reveal their personality disposition. On test date, the wife revealed need for dependence, affection and attention—particularly from representative figures in life. A need for polygamy was evident in the husband. This was further substantiated through GSR fluctuations. As just mentioned above, during counselling the husband showed lots of resistances to cooperate—particularly in disclosing matters related to his libidinal urges and his level of satisfaction. As in marital relationship this is one of the significant reasons for disharmony, and his very highly defensive nature raised doubt in the counsellor and it was felt necessary to probe more into this issue. On subsequent sessions it could be revealed that the man has had an illicit relation with his elder brother's wife. He has been controlled throughout by that woman, so much so that, in several occasions, he did not hesitate to insult his wife in front of others. Thus, depth interpretation helped him to realise after a long time that he has become easily irritable in his interaction with his wife and started accusing her on petty matters with a desire to shift all blame onto her. In actuality, he wanted her to leave him which will enable him to be more close with that woman (elder brother's wife).

The question of his getting married in spite of having a desire for such illicit relation (of which he is conscious as he had been involved with that woman since long) has been taken-up in the counselling process. The wife was also counselled on the matters related to her personality predisposition and also to learn why she was feeling so much shattered even to face a fact that her husband was involved in illicit relation.

From the above examples, it is clear that counselling can provide the couple insight into each other's personality which in turn inculcates in them a need to share, and also a sense of commitment, trust and responsibility to each other.

Marriage Counselling : Indian Scenario

In marriage counselling ordinarily the partners appear with a single problem, namely, adjustment problems with in-laws, or disagreements between the partners in deciding over the methods to be implemented in upbringing their child, or about the child's schooling, and so on. Gradually during the subsequent sessions lot of other problems came to the surface, all of which are mostly the offshoots of the above. Problems can be derooted only when the counsellor becomes aware of the process as to how the problems got enrooted. Of course, precipitating events need to be elicited and dealt with accordingly. Thereupon predisposing factors be taken over consideration because prevention is no less important than intervention. Otherwise, counselling will turn out to be a method of symptomatic amelioration of the problems reported; the inevitable outcome of which would be recurrence of the symptoms in future.

Precipitating events would cover—on the one hand, individual factors of both the partners, and on the other, environmental factors. Both of these are likely to contribute to their present problems. Some of the individual factors are, gap between level of aspiration and degree of attainment, attitude towards parenthood, major conflicts in life and coping strategies employed, sex conflict, sexual problems and guilt, and attitudinal differences between the couple (detailed later). Environmental factors may be in the nature of employment of the partners, time they can spend for each other and in also for the family, chronic illness in the family, illness of the life partner, and its prognosis, financial crisis in the family (detailed later).

Precipitating : Common Precursors

(1) Disclosure of the previous affairs, or marriage leading to an apprehension of infidelity. (2) Change in job and/or unemployment after marriage. (3) Employment of the wife after marriage (in some cases in Indian culture it causes problem). (4) Infertility, bisexual or homosexual lifestyle, diminished or excessive sex drive in one of the partners which the other cannot cope with (Buxton, 1991). The latter is equally important in Indian clients as well.

Separation Anxiety : Parents in the Indian culture, by and large, expect that their offsprings will provide them the opportunity to select their match. In case of love marriage, parents feel that they have been deprived of such right of theirs. Being frustrated and disappointed they sometimes do not mind even to abandon the couple from their house and their property enjoyment rights. Such a feeling of separation acts as a precursor for family disharmony. Even in arranged marriage, girls, in this culture, usually have a feeling of separation from their family of origin; at the same time, girls take long time to adjust with the in-laws' life style, causes distress in the in-law's' family, and more particularly in the interaction process of the newly married couple. Husband and other members of the family may lose patience and start commenting on the girl's attitude adversely. However, separation related stress has been reported by Cameron *et al*, (1998) in the West also.

Parenting : Problems involving parenting are disagreement over procreation. In India, couples are ordinarily much concerned about the time period that lapses between their marriage and arrival of the first child. In older days—couple used to take longer time to plan for first child. In recent years, though there seems to prevail an idea of having a child within a couple of years, sometimes disagreement is reported on this issue between the couple. Also, disagreement is reported in Indian culture regarding the gender of the child. Such gender preference is dangerous. Many a times it causes serious stress in their life adjustment, to the extent of neglecting the child (of unpreferred gender), and in some cases even abandonment of the wife. A female engineer reported that her husband abandoned her along with her baby since he heard that he has been the father of a female baby. Finally, this has led to separation in them (husband also is an engineer). Crisis is also evident between the couple for the management of adolescents progeny (Cameron *et al*, 1998) both in the East and the West. But method of management varies a lot over culture.

Soon after child birth, and thereupon when the child starts schooling, in some cases, the couple experience severe distress in redefining the structure of the relationship—particularly with regard to sharing responsibilities. This is more acute when the wife is also equally educated and employed. In traditional Indian system, job outside the family boundary has not been a designated role for the woman. As such, many senior members of the family, and even many modern husbands do not prefer women to pursue higher education and occupation after marriage. Resistance is shown not only with regard to the woman's pursuing office job, but with regard to their professional consultation also, namely, medical practice for physician wife in some occasions. Obviously, such highly qualified women become totally disappointed after marriage. Such a negative attitude of the family members, particularly of the husband(s), further fuels the distress the women otherwise experiences in their family interaction. On the other hand, it is also often reported that some of the women who have consented to hold independent service, face a sort of non-cooperation from the in-laws which causes attitudinal differences between the husband and the wife with respect to their occupational positions, financial status, sharing of each other's income in family budget, and so on. Issues concerning reconciliation of the traditional Indian social values and norms with those of the modern trends have become some of the major source of stress in life style of the couples. The above-mentioned factors are more severe in India, as joint family structure is mostly prevailing here even now. Of course it doesn't mean that the joint family does not have its advantages. It has very many contributions in the family—particularly in the upbringing of the children. It is a value clash between the older generation and modern youth, however, that takes place in respect to their style of life namely, dress, habits, attitudes, interaction patterns, pursing occupation, higher education, responsibility sharing, cohesiveness, and so on.

Such attitudinal differences are to be taken care of in the counselling sessions. Both of the couple require analyses of their deep rooted personality complexes, namely, inferiority, suspiciousness, inadequacy, need for supremacy, extreme dependency, and so on. It is also required, in some instances, that senior members of the family, too, praticipate jointly in counselling sessions. Unfortunately, seniors mostly disagree to participate; more strikingly, very often one of the couple shows strong resistance to receive counselling services. If, on request from the partner, he/she gets ready to comply with, shortly refrains from continuing such sessions. Thus the counsellor's attempt to conduct counselling sessions adequately remains incomplete, as the counsellor has to depend on the mercy of the absentee. However, marriage counselling in such cases turns out to be an individual counselling concerning related problems.

Environmental Factors

Joint family system though has some advantages, particularly in the upbringing of the children and sharing responsibilities, nowadays it appears that couples report that disadvantages overpower its advantage. This is primarily due to attitudinal differences between the modern couple and their in-laws. Expectations of the in-laws from their daughter-in-laws are different in our culture compared to those of the others. This is because, in Indian culture, the role of spouse is rigidly designed. In-laws, in some cases, are found reluctant to relax the designated boundary of such predetermined roles of spouses, no matter whether their daughter-in-law is employed or housewife. Wives, nowadays, usually expect their husband to share with them the family responsibilities, namely, household matters. Some men, particularly those with conservative mentality and those who want to retain the orthodox traditional Indian system, are found reluctant to share such activities with their life partners. Because traditionally such participation of the men with their wives was not granted as a designed role of men. In some cases, in the modern era, men are willing to share such responsibilities with their wives, but due to their non-assertive personality trait as against family disapproval they fail to get involved in such matters directly, though psychologically they want to share. This is because they think that their parents with traditional mentality will not consent to it. Such husbands are in dilemma whether to share with their wives or to lose the support of their parents. This causes strong anguish in the wife it the husband finally refrains from sharing such activities.

Coming to the other side of the coin, when the husbands want their wives to assume major responsibilities, some women fail to assume such role. This is because they have been brought up with such assumption that some such roles are beyond the designated roles of woman in Indian culture. They, because of their dependent nature, refrain from taking such responsibilities, even though their husbands desire so. This causes anguish in the males, particularly in a nuclear family set-up. As against this, some of the females want to overpower males, but males do not approve. These are some of the examples as to how negotiating a division of labour (sharing) between the newly married couple in a family fails. Though cultural factors are partly responsible for such disharmony, personality characteristics of the couple are found to be more important as determinants in causing such problems of adjustment. Such problems prompt us to look for some predisposing factors in the personality of the couples; many a times the in-laws too need to be counselled. But strong resistance is noted in both the parties.

Predisposing personality characteristics of the couple mostly reveal :

Problems are in communication, commitment, autonomy and attachment. Problems related to trust, responsibility, assertiveness, decision-making. Also—and perhaps the most important ones—are those related to the unconscious matrix of the relationship (Karpel, 1994) which includes, to name a few—new need to depend, need to dominate, fear of rejection, sexuality, and so on. All these are to be considered in the counselling sessions to develop an adequate understanding between the couple.

Some prerequisites to choose the members of the group

The counsellor must have adequate insight to choose group members so that the purpose of such arrangement is not lost altogether. The counsellor has to keep in mind certain assumptions group counselling is based on. The counsellor has to be sure about the basic latent potentialities of the client so that he/she can—Share individual problems, can be concerned about the other group members, can developed trust on others, and also can be trusted by others, can learn from group interaction to the extent of taking responsibility to change himself/herself.

In sum : There are lots of commonness between individual counselling and group counselling. Both aim to help the client achieve a mental state of self-evaluation, self-acceptance, and self-direction. But differences are also evident. Unlike the group method where the client may have solace from the awareness that there are others with similar problems like that of his/her, in individual method he/she can't share his/her problem with clients. Accordingly, in group method, he/she can learn from his/her interaction with group members, while in individual method his/her interaction is limited in one-to-one relationship (with the counsellor only). Group set-up has been found to be most effective in vocational counselling, educational counselling, career choice counselling, etc. Individual counselling is effective, as mentioned earlier, with persons having deep rooted psychological problems (unconscious conflicts), persons with psychosomatic tendencies, disruptive adolescents with defiant attitude to the authority figure etc. Group counselling must not be considered as a substitute for individual counselling. Nevertheless, an integration of group method with individual method of counselling has been found effective in many instances.

Chapter 15

DILEMMA IN COUNSELLING : INDIAN PERSPECTIVE

Background Information

Culture plays an extremely significant role in an individual's development—in defining his/her inner self as well as in determining the constituents of his/her perception of the external reality. As already mentioned in the previous chapters there are fundamental differences among the Eastern and the Western social life style and culture. Such divergent concepts of the self, the society, and that of the culture highlight the need for developing culture-specific counselling (even psychotherapeutic) paradigms. One of the reasons for repeated failure in counselling outcome may be because of our rigid application of the Western models in our cultural set-up. Discontentment has been voiced by the clinicians and academicians (Patel, 2000), on the application of Westernised explanatory concepts of counselling/psychotherapy to Indian context.

A clinician's expertise for assessments and intervention planning can best be understood only when the clinician can recognise the cognitive developmental orientations of the client. Having understood the primary and secondary cognitive developmental orientations, the clinicians face problems in convincing the client about its significance in the manifestation of behavioural pathology. Culturally sensitive issues ingrained in the clients' cognitive-structure raises strong resistance to break through, and also to realise that restructuring (modification) of such cognitive developmental orientations would no way make the client debarred from social acceptance. Many of these clients though have access of modified cognitive, emotional, and behavioural resources inherent in them through several interactions, in counselling session mostly they tend to rely on primary orientations only to understand their specific issues under discussion. Primary orientations are net results of societal upbringing since childhood.

Sources of Dilemma

Parental upbringing

Age of the Client : Childhood : Childhood experiences are most crucial in understanding psychopathology of symptoms manifested later in life. Such experiences create deep rooted seats in the mind of the child with varieties of tentacles, which the child retains for his whole life through disturbed and unhappy adolescence and young adulthood. That is why the present write-up will focus primarily upon the problems which begin in childhood but become apparent mostly in adolescence and young adulthood. It would be better, I think, to consider the major developmental stages of cognitive development as advocated by Piaget (1985). In fact, clinicians with development counselling orientation do prefer to consider Piaget's viewpoint of cognitive development, namely sensory-motor, situational, reflective, and dialectic. For detail the reader is referred to Piaget (1985) and Rigazio-Digilio *et al*, (1997). Each of these orientations involves a complexity of language but ultimately represents the 'meaning making process', of the client (Rigazio-Digilio *et al*, 1997). Cognitive developmental stages may be universal but ultimately representation of meaning to the life events varies across culture. Meaning representation is largely an outcome of childhood learning which one receives through parental upbringing. Let us examine now some of the problems we frequently come across with our adolescents and young adults during counselling sessions.

Age of the client : Adolescence : The most remarkable characteristics of adolescence is change (in physiological, psychological and social spares) so much so that it cause stress and strain in them. But Margaret Mead (1953) long back reported that adolescence, by itself, is not necessarily a period of stress and turmoil, unless the social pattern and life style determining factors make adolescents stressed. Thus, e.g., social considerations and determining pattern of thought, behaviour, of the Western societies need not necessarily hold good in Indian societies. Sociologists and anthropologists of the East are of the opinion that adolescence is a 'cultural invention' (Rao, 1981).

Volumes are available on the various problems of adolescence, still our knowledge about Indian adolescents seem to be incomplete. There are wide cross-cultural variations in the onset of adolescence. In Finland, some girls start menstruating as early as 9 yrs. In our culture, menarche starts, on an average, between 12 to 14 yrs (Das & Chattopadhyay, 1982). The onset of adolescence for the boys of our culture, as revealed through ANS and CNS measures, was found to be 12 yrs, and the duration of adolescence, as measured through physiological stress factors, extended up to 12-17 yrs, with a peak of anxiety and adjustment problems around 15-16 yrs, whereas, on endocrinological measures, namely, testosterone, prolactin and cortisol, the peak anxiety was evident around age 11-12 yrs. Associated other measures, like tooth age, bone age, etc. corroborated well with the physiological and biochemical measures (Mallick, Ghosh, and Chattopadhyay, 1986), though in some cases subjective measures of stress failed to corroborate with those of the objective measures. The latter discrepancies may be attributed to the limitations of the subjects in revealing their exact feelings onto the questionnaire measures (Mitra, Bandyopadhyay & Chattopadhyay, 2002).

Epidemiological studies in India have given prevalence rate of psychological problems which are about 2-30% amongst adolescents (Bhola and Kapur, 2000) of which more than 8% prevalence is of psychological disturbances in general, and nearly 6% prevalence of emotional disturbances were reported amongst boys (Sinha and Kapur, 2001; Kapur, Rao and Dalal, 1994). A higher prevalence rate of emotional problems (10.9%) amongst girls was evident (Gaur, Murthy, and Nathawat, 2001). About 1.5 million Brown Sugar addicts (12% females) was reported (Sinha and Kapur, 2001). By this time the above mentioned problems have increased both in frequency and in degree. But unfortunately public initiation to provide adequate clinical support has not been proportionate to the gravity of the situation. Reluctance to come for consultation appears to be more prominent in the parents, when the problem is in relation to their female children.

Gender differences and attitude toward parents

Gender differences prevail amongst adolescents in India with regard to their attitudes toward parents. Mother is ordinarily perceived as more punitive than father, still mother is the major source of affection, mostly for the boys (Paintal and Pandey, 1996). Of course, variations are also noted. Many a times adolescents perceive father as more punitive and become relatively more free to mother. Attitudinal differences are also markedly present in some parts of India amongst parents in providing educational and occupational facilities to the girls. However, the issue of gender discrimination has not been that significant, particularly in urban set-up, as because girls are no longer debarred from such facilities now. Gender discriminations in some other perspective come to the surface even in the urban set-up (see Chapter on Group Counselling). However, most adolescents suffer from 'identity crisis', because they are neither entrusted with adult responsibilities (though they demand for) nor are they treated as children. Such an amorphous position in social interdependence causes confusion and feelings of alienation. With such a mental state they step in young adulthood. The counsellor has to balance between the two, i.e., adolescents' needs and demands, and parental attitudinal differences. The counsellor has to remain important to the client as well as to their parents.

Striking gender differences in adolescents symptomatology have been clinically observed. Girls have a proclivity towards internally turned symptoms (such as anxiety, depression, somatisation) whereas for the boys conduct disorders, hyperactivity, attentional difficulties, school refusals have been reported (Bhola and Kapur, 2000; Ollendick and King, 1994). Poor academic achievement associated with sex guilt, negative social interaction, OCD, somatic complaints, self-harm, (to the extent of suicide) are frequent in adolescents in India irrespective of gender (Sinha and Kapur, 2001; Kar, Pandey, Mishra, Sengupta and Das, 1996). Loneliness, depression (Sanyal, 2004), poor self-concept, examination phobia (Sinha, 2000; Rao and Partha Sarathi, 1993; Bhaduri, Upamanyu and Goyel, 2000) are also reported quite often in our adolescents. These information are important in formulating counselling programmes for the adolescents of Indian culture. Because many a times, the goal setting in counselling and parental attitude in accepting that goal which deems suitable for the client clinically do not go hand in hand. Thus, clinical needs and social demands appear at variance with each other.

Attitude towards sex

Attitude towards sex amongst our people is quite different from that of the West. Sex related matters have bee perceived, by the orthodox Indian society, as something to be suppressed. Its expression in any form, namely, through group discussion or free mixing paticularly for the adolescents and the youths, used to be prohibited throughout. Such an attitude prevails even now in many senior people of India. Verbal expression of sex-oriented thoughts even amongst peers is considered by them as violation of the cultural norms. As free mixing with the persons of the opposite sex has not been permissible, parents of our adolescents become highly apprehensive thinking of the possible consequences if their offsprings violate such rules. They become excessively vigilant about each movement and curious about every action of their offsprings. Such inspectionism, in turn, causes lots of adjustment problems in both the young and the old. Recently, through media, adolescents are exposed to certain scenes, which they interpret in their own way as because they can't clarify their doubts and curiosities. Mostly such suppressed information produces guilt in them, which prevails even late in their life and causes several problems in their academic and social spheres of life. These information are essential while formulating counselling programme for the adolescents for our culture. Counsellor has to balance between the two orthogonal views of the young and the old in counselling sessions. Whom to educate first in the counselling session, the adolescents (to refrain from sex) or the old (to restructure their cognition considering the technological advancements, and socio-cultural changes over time)? Unless a balance can be maintained between the adolescents and their parents, counselling in unidimensional direction will be of no use. Because, our adolescents and youths do not stay separately from their parents. They have to have daily life interactions with each other.

Vignettes of some of the adolescent cases highlighting the conflicts generated from societal norms

Case I : A girl (14+ yrs) of a middle class socio-economic status, studying at Class VIII, only child, both parents working, comes with the complaints of feeling of loneliness, helplessness and history of attempted suicide (thrice) with a total duration of two years. Rigidity and stubbornness also noted. Intermittent pharmacological treatment was reported but never had undergone psychological intervention. On enquiry, it could be revealed that nagging parents with traditional mentality (to the extent that the client was not allowed to use wrist watch on right hand), used to compare the child with others for academic achievement. Information about sex couldn't be revealed in initial sessions. Induced anxiety out of academic competitions, and fear of failure leading to suicidal attempts and sex related conflicts are perhaps some of the typical complaints of such age groups of clients in our culture.

Case II : A male student of Class XII (18 yrs), middle class family background, father employed, mother housewife, one younger brother, comes with the complaints of lack of concentration in studies, irritability, lack of confidence, self-image highly negative; total duration though since long, problems aggravated for last 1 yr. On enquiry revealed ambivalent attitude towards his mother, mostly dependent on his father (who stays abroad for service), and lots of conflicts and confusions about sex since 12+ yrs. No formal psychiatric treatment received so far. This is his first visit for psychological consultation.

Case III : A boy (15 yrs) of Class IX standard, younger of the 2 siblings (elder sister married), belongs to a family where his father has taken voluntary retirement and mother is a housewife, comes with the complaints of easy distractability while studying absentmindedness, irritability, shyness, tendency to lie, nervousness, misuse of money, lack of interest in games, but addiction to TV, total duration—3 yrs. On enquiry it could be revealed that difference of opinion prevails with parents regarding appointment of many private tutors (parents want more number of teachers), lack of attention and emotional attachment from parents, and being teased by classmates due to his social inhibitions; can't take part in discussion with peers on several day-to-day matters including sex related matters. Has not received any formal psychiatric treatment; was brought by the parents for psychological intervention.

Case IV : A male student of 1st year engineering (19+ yrs), has one elder sister (PG student), comes from upper-middle class family, father is in service and mother is a housewife. Reported—difficulties in adjustment with college friends, not satisfied with the present stream of his education, which he has been assigned during counselling by the experts of the joint entrance examination; depressed; occasional self-talk (reported by the parents), aggressiveness, fear of failure since last 6 months; has been on pharmacotherapy for last 6 months. Slight improvement but not satisfied; has come for psychological intervention for first time. On enquiry revealed—feelings of superiority but poor self-assessment; sentimental, too much fantasy bound, lack of determination (but high need to achieve), received discouragement from his parents, fault finding tendency with others, indecisive and doubtful about endurance of his love affair (at this stage the counsellor not sure whether it is one-sided love). On the one hand depends on parents (but this need is not fulfilled) and on the other, desires to establish relation with a girl though lacks confidence in this; wants parents' approval (underlying need) for affair, but afraid of parents' rejection in this regard (cultural norm).

Carryover effects of parental over protection

Age of the clients : youth : Adolescents growing into adults have to learn to relate themselves with the other members of the society and also to reciprocate accordingly. Such an apparently matter-of-fact issue is not really so in our culture. Sometimes it appears otherwise also. This is because up to this stage of their life our adolescents are sometimes debarred from taking active role in any sort of decision-making process, and in most cases they are debarred from even sharing their views, in some major issues in life, with the senior. Becoming independent would, ipso facto, mean becoming responsible for one's own decisions and actions in different spheres of life. viz., economic, occupational, social, etc. But many a time it is reported that the youths in our culture become easily emotionally shattered and high strung, when they are assigned to such responsibilities. This is because they have so far been shielded totally under parental guidance, supervision; such dependency interferes with their independent way of exerting one's own power when necessary. Sudden pressure, e.g., when in occupational set-up, to be independent in decision-making becomes highly stressful and sometimes even painful for these youngsters.

The other related issues comprise of apprehension whether it would be possible to make normal sexual adjustment, whether it would be possible to secure a placement that will be absorbing and inspiring; whether would be able to work independently but individually to obtain a desired social status.

In sum : In many instances, parental over-protection since childhood is later perceived by the adolescents and the youths as interference in their normal development of self-confidence and development of general attitude for self-help.

Vignettes of some cases : youth

Case I : Young adult, 21 yrs., B.E. III yr student, got involved with a girl of about his same age, who is a student of B.Sc. As neighbours since their childhood, both of them had opportunities to interact with each other initially as peers and gradually during adolescence they fell in love with each other. Both the families also has consent to their affairs (in Indian culture family consent provides a strong security for the youths to materialised affair) with an expectation of marriage after completion of the formal education. Up to this age of life, they reported to have experienced severe contradictions in decision-making regarding their future on several occasions; they also experienced contradictions regarding some of their present life style, so much so that they themselves took initiative to come for pre-marital counselling together. Interview revealed that the girl was highly possessive, whilst the boy was meekly submissive, with poor decision-making ability; the latter has been dependent on his parents throughout for taking decisions on major life issues. In different occasions their confrontations crystallised to that extent that in an individual session the boy disclosed his unwillingness to marry the girl because of her stubbornness and possessive attitudes. He confessed confidentially "Please help me doctor to get rid of this girl... I won't marry her but I can't confess this to her, because she might then commit suicide." The girl, on the other hand, in an individual session confessed that "Please see that we get married soon; I can't think of any other man except this guy in my life...; though, of late, he has been showing irritation and aggression towards me on many occasions, I love him really." They boy realised that the girl, with such an attitude won't be able to stay with his parents in a joint family set-up. The girl, infact, insisted upon having a separate establishment after marriage. Separation from his parents due to marriage is unimaginable to the boy, he felt very much perturbed with her proposal. The boy has been brought up throughout in joint family structure, whilst the girl has been brought up in nuclear family set-up.

Case II : A female doctor, MBBS, 28 yrs, got married to an engineer, B.E., 30 yrs; arranged marriage. After 2 yrs of marriage both came for counselling, with wife's initiative. Their complaints—(i) the man is highly possessed by his mother to that extent that it disturbs their private life (reported by the wife). The man cannot contradict his mother in setting their regular life style (mother's interference). (ii) During negotiation of this marriage, though the parents of the husband agreed to allow their daughter-in-law to continue her medical practice, soon after marriage they resisted such practice so strongly that they have not allowed her to examine and treat patients at her own residence either (question of going out of the residence for medical practice did not arise). The wife was not only surprised but shocked too for such an abrupt change of her in-laws' attitude towards her profession. She perceived it as a breach of contract and expected her husband to take initiative to mitigate it—but all in vain. The wife came for counselling first, and, after a few sessions, insisted upon her husband to join at least for individual sessions. The husband came reluctantly two times only just to comply with his wife, apparently. Finally, he declined to report as because he did not want to be exposed to the counsellor that he fails to assert in taking his role as a husband. This problem of the husband is more acute if he has to encounter his mother, which he has never done before.

Case III : Engineer couple, in their late 20s, both employed at the same corporate organisation, married for last 2 yrs (love marriage), came for counselling intervention with the complaints that the girl has been facing non-cooperation from the in-laws. The girl thus wants a separate establishment, whilst her husband declines this proposal. So much so that the husband has given threat of divorce while the wife resists it stating 'marriage does not intent divorce'. As such, the wife strongly resists the husband's proposal. The husband was found to be a variable in sticking to his decision of living with his parents as because he has purchased a separate apartment to live with his wife only, but sometimes resists to go over there. Though the wife took the initiative to come for counselling, the husband was not at all willing. The husband came only twice very reluctantly on request from his wife. The wife describes her husband as 'Mom's son'. She reported that her husband tells lies and is manipulative too. 'He realises that injustice has been done on me, but wants me to tolerate it. I can't bear it any more. But I don't want divorce.'

Case IV : A woman divorcee of about 30 yrs, MBA, employed (temporary basis) in a corporate organisation, married (love marriage) to an accountant (2nd marriage), of about 27 yrs, M. Com., employed in another corporate organisation. Initial 2 yrs their relationship was reported to be very good. Later contradictions, confrontations, developed in decision-making so much so that they consulted a legal practitioner (separately), and finally prior to filing a divorce case, came, for counselling as a last resort. This was predominantly the wife's decision to take counsellor's assistance. Since, for both the partners, it was second marriage, family people showed non-co-operation, as in India, such marriage is not encouraged—particularly by the seniors of the family (situation, of late is changing as the senior members of the family are now showing some change in attitude; of course many a times even now a strong resistance is noticed from many in this regard). Secondly, unhappiness prevailed in the family as because the wife was senior to the husband by age, which is not customary in Indian culture. Thirdly, during interview the wife complained of her husband's loose character. They have had no issue till now (5 yrs of marriage). The husband was reluctant to come for counselling; visited only 3 times and reported that he dislikes his wife's domineering and aggressive behaviour. In the meantime, the husband arranged for a transfer of his service (with an intention to stay separately, disclosed during interview) though gave an impression to his wife that this transfer was pre-scheduled for him. The wife, on the contrary, was suspicious about the intentions of his transfer due to his previous objectionable behaviours, like e-mail chatting with many girls to the extent of promiscuity. During interview though some such negative qualities of her husband were highlighted by the wife, she too had shown inconsistency in her reaction patterns to him. For example, out of aggression, several times she had not replied to his telephone calls, refrained frome-mail contact with her husband, and so on, at times, particularly at night, when she used to feel very lonely, used to initiate e-mail chatting with her husband intermittently. The husband used to take advantage of such weakness and consequent incongruent behaviour of his wife (wife felt exploited, still failed to control her impulse to contact her husband at times). During interview, she used to say several times "... if I leave my husband, he will go astray; doctor, can I sacrifice my life enjoyment to save the life of this man who was initially so good?" "... As I am a divorcee, i wouldn't like to go for a divorce second time." Again, she used to say, "I would like to give him a lesson legally."

Case V : MBSS, 3rd yr female, student, 22 yrs, only child of a middle class family came with the complaint of lack of concentration in studies so much so that when she had to appear for supplementary examination while clearing 2nd yr medical, she became irritable, had disturbed interaction with friends. Depth inerviews in later sessions revealed strong inferiority, fear of rejection by the persons of the opposite sex; has taken academic help from a classmate who wants private relation, the client expressed unwillingness, though feels strong need to receive his assistance for her academic pursuit. Further analysis revealed that the client, because of family pressure, refrains to maintain relationship with the boy, though she has developed a positive feeling towards the boy. The clients' decision to continue relationship with her boy friend, will make her parents severely depressed—this is what the girl was concerned with when she came for counselling. Her dilemma was—whether to accept that guy or to leave her parents.

Case VI : A graduate male, 33 yrs. Only son of a middle class family, employed, got involved with a girl of 23 yrs for last 10 yrs since when he used to coach the girl privately for her academic pursuit. Parents of the client expressed their unwillingness to the girl of her being entangled with their son, and they advised their son to stop private tuition. Parents resisted this relationship, mainly because of age gap between the would-be couple and also because of difference in family standards. The client (male) came for counselling. Parents were called for. Mother agreed to come but father didn't.

In sum : Problems of youth may broadly be categorised as—

- Motivational (lack of interest, lack of ambition and achievement, etc.),
- Emotional (excessive anxiety, very high drive but lack of confidence, immaturity, hypersensitivity, shyness, withdrawal, etc.),
- Moral (guilt out of excessive lying, stealing, becoming unruly, and matters related to virility, virginity, and so on).

Adolescents and youths who are confused and fail to take right decision, counselling is to help them to clarify their conflicts and confusions; to help them develop adequate self-esteem and self-confidence, so as to enable them to make the right decisions. Indian studies (e.g., Rao, 1964, 1965a,b, 1967a,b, 1969, 1970, 1971, 1972, 1973 and 1974) have long before emphasised the need for counselling of our adolescents and young adults in their perspective.

Please refer to the Case III of the above vignettes, where both the couple during initial interview and later during intervention have expressed about their feelings in a divergent manner. Both have expressed some positive qualities of their partners, though negative feelings did overweigh those positive qualities. However, relatively more fluctuations in thoughts and actions were evident in the wife (flexible access). Such flexibility, indeed, causes problems in intervention sessions too.

When we refer to Case IV of the vignettes, we find that the couple gave a diffused orientation to their problem, particularly with the wife. Her presentation of problems was haphazard throughout. Such inconsistency in feeling/emotion, and action, i.e., a multiple perspective, make the counsellor confused about the selection of intervention strategy. However, a skilful counsellor may utilise such diversity in thought as resources of the client; these resources may be best utilised in cognitive restructuring of the clients in a better way than of those clients who have one rigid fixed orientation.

Also a close scrutiny of such cases, who apparently present a multiple orientation in reporting their complaints, (may be to maintain a desired face-value to the counsellor, or to make the counsellor confused) finally show a bend towards a definite orientation (requires high skills of the part of the counsellor to get it revealed through the client), in attributing meaning to their life events/experiences. A clinician has to be very careful and attentive in detecting such a bend of the client and also to decide upon when when cognitive restructuring would be required therapeutically. For example, a male, 24 yrs, graduate (engineer), unmarried, employed, came for consultation with major complaints of OCD (repeated hand washing, checking-rechecking). During counselling, when he has helped to associate his present discomfort with his past life events and experiences, he was rigidly focussing his father's very strict and domineering personality and lack of emotional bondage he has had with his father. He also, during intervention session, expressed that he lacks the capacity to exercise logic appropriately in decision-making. 'I am overpowered by emotion,' the client said. But he took a considerable long time to express his experience of sex with his sister-in-law though could associate later during the session the impact of such an event onto his present complaints. He then reported that his academic progress started deteriorating ever since he got involved sexually with his sister-in-law. He can't accept such an interaction with his sister-in-law logically, though emotionally he has failed to control in refraining himself from such relation. This shows that of the two significant life events the client narrated, more focussed was his father's personality and life interaction with him. The less focussed one, i.e., his sex-related guilt, got expressed very late during the sessions. Thus, the client had one fixed orientation towards his problems, i.e., sexual guilt, though he was trying to cover it in the beginning through his father's attitude towards him. Apparently the client was trying to make his father responsible for his present problems. Indeed such attitude of his father has significant impact onto his personality development; may be that his desire to get involved into illicit sex was a compensatory mechanism on his part. That is, to prove to himself that he can move on by his own beyond his father's ruling, as and when he desire so. This, of course, required detailed discussion during counselling. The client though admitted such compensatory mechanism, took long time to resolve his sex guilt. In actuality, shifting blame towards his father was a defence on his part. He was trying to justify his misdeed with such a plea. But later realised during the session that unless one has got inclination, one cannot get involved into such an action, no matter whether adverse circumstances may instigate him for the same. This indeed requires capacity to control emotion adequately. At this juncture the client cited several other incidents and experiences of his life and said "Doctor, I'm throughout emotionally overpowered; I understand, I need to be controlled by logic, but I fail". What makes one emotionally overpowered, that too was discussed with the client in subsequent sessions.

A clinician-counsellor has to have that efficiency which would help him/her to determine clearly the primary and secondary cognitive, emotional, and behavioural orientations of the client toward his/her presenting problems for which the clients seek intervention. Once the counsellor is sure about the client's such frame of references, then it is up to the counsellor to decide upon when to encourage vertical movement, and when horizontal—in reframing the client's orientation through psychological intervention, if required.

A word of caution : Untrained counsellors are likely to cause severe harm in the client in introducing such a shift in cognitive frame of the client.

Influence of media to emulate the culture

Youths in the modern era are exposed to several conflicting and stressful situation. Owing to their exposure to other cultural phenomena and events through mass media, magazines, and through internet, they are often tempted to imitate and emulate other modes and patterns of behaviour not acceptable to our traditional norms and values. Also, owing to several political and socio-economic factors, a significant section of our youth is becoming estranged and alienated from society. For some youths, their revolt against traditional social norms is expressed through unrest, whilst, for some others, it is found in their resort to drug abuse, espousal of other culture(s), etc. They appear to be increasingly groping for a meaning in life consonant with their own ideas and expectations. They appear to be neither acculturated nor fully encultured because they become tempted to intermingle different cultural norms at a time.

Religion

In India, many people, even today, when under emotional distress, visit religious centres irrespective of the religion one believes in. The religious institutions/places as such seem to have power of healing (Raghuram, Venkateswaram, Ramkrishnan and Weiss, 2002), and their leaders provide them emotional support, and when necessary prescribe antidotes, indigenous in nature (e.g., sacred flower, oil, water, roots of plants, etc.); the latter has placebo impact in the distressed. In a survey in Tamil Nadu (South India), Campion and Bhugra (1996) found that about 45% of the psychiatric patients consulted a religious leader before attending the hospitals. Owing to brevity of space, it is not possible to provide here a detailed description of all varieties of traditional healing methods being practice in India, but adequate research evidences are available to justify the positive impact of such methods in helping the distressed residing in different parts of India. A counsellor has to have a clear idea about a given client's religious bend, if any, and nature of religious resources the client is used to receive before.

Bend towards medical model of prescription

By and large people in this country believe in medical model of treatment. While consulting a physician, as they get a prescription and physician-patient relationship is retained through the prescription, at the end of the counselling session too, our clients mostly assume that they will be provided with a prescription similar to that of a medical practitioner. Sometimes they enquire astonishingly, that how treatment can be continued without a medical prescription? Of course, it must not mean that medical model of treatment has no importance. Quite a good number of psychiatric patients require pharmacotherapy, and a good number of clients require pharmacotherapy as a secondary aid, while they are on counselling. The author's intention here is to focus on our clients' attitude, which is largely medical prescription bound. From the point of view, religious leaders also can satisfy very well their clients' need to possess a prescription, whilst the psychologist-counsellors cannot (it is totally based on verbal give and take). This causes a dilemma in our clients mostly. A counsellor does prescribe but in the form of homework, and other related methods, but not in the form of medicine. Our clients mostly confined the term prescription in context to medicine only. This is because treatment and medicine vis-a-vis treatment and prescription is very much in congruence with their cognitive orientation.

Dilemma

In 1973, two models of psychotherapy were reported by Neki, namely, 'Guru-Chela' (teacher-people) relationship, and the 'Sahaja' therapy (togetherness). The former was considered ideal for Indian patients (the term 'patient' has been used by Prof. Neki), as because teacher-taught relationship implies that one (the pupil) can be made knowledgeable with assistance from the other (the teacher), while the latter implies sharing responsibilities. The former has become more suitable in Indian set-up, probably because Indian family upbringing style induces a feeling of dependency onto the senior/superior, particularly in decision making tasks. Such a need to depend, as a cultural ingredient, raises expectation in the clients to remain passive even in deciding upon the suitable means to reach his/her life goal, through solving problems, for which he seeks counselling services. Such a dependency causes a lots of problems in the initial-phase—namely, transference related problems, and also during the termination (of intervention programmes). Counsellors, in India, have to be specially alert in handling the consequences which might arise from such typical attitude of the clients.

Dilemma 1 : When clients' expectation from the counsellor contradicts the counselling norms

When our clients prepare themselves to receive assistance from either a religious leader or from a medical practitioner, or from a clinical psychologist/counsellor, they are very well ensured from within (though no professional, be he a religious person, or a medical, para-medical practitioner, encourage the clients to depend on him/her) that they can depend on the respective professional. When the clients start taking medicine (be it indigenous or otherwise), they become automatically dependent on medicine so much so that many a times it comes to our notice that they go on continuing the same medicine either regularly or even sporadically without consulting the physician intermittently. Picture is totally different in case of counselling, where they don't find any other object or person to depend on, but the counsellor (exceptions are noted where the clients want to get rid of medicine and to be treated by other means. But number of such clients are relatively less). Contrary to their expectation, the counsellor has to encourage the client and enable him/her to learn how to be self-dependent. While formulating counselling model we need to bear this in our mind. Indian child rearing practices and family interaction style, by and large, does not encourage autonomy and independence in decision-making, whilst in the West, these are considered as positive qualities of a child. To a certain extent decisions are culturally determined in India. Though situation is changing over time, there too, youngsters are taking hasty decisions in certain spheres of their life, which, in turn, make the problem further acute. Therefore, in Indian model of counselling, the counsellor has to be careful whether approach like that of Roger's ('person centred') would really help the client, at least initially, when the client, normally, would expect the counsellor to guide him directly. Of course, it must not mean that whatever the client would demand the counsellor has to comply with. This causes another dilemma in the counselling session.

Dilemma 2 : (i) The basic admonition of counselling, in the real sense of the term, does not permit the counsellor to impose his/her values, and thoughts, and decisions onto the client;

(ii) The counsellor realises very well that the client's basic need to depend requires modification to ensure enhancement of self-esteem later;

(iii) The counsellor understands that, finally, the client has to learn and implement the methods by himself/herself to root out his/her problems; however,

(iv) Initial non-directive approach makes the client disappointed (as this approach takes little more times to elicit information) as he wants immediate relief from his distress : (a) does not understand the lasting effect of the intervention; or (b) fails to bear with patience the duration required to root out the problem.

(v) If the client discontinues sessions being frustrated with the counsellor's non-directive approach (client's demand, though not correct) it causes further harm to the client as symptoms would aggravate;

(vi) If the counsellor decides upon directive approach, there too the counsellor experiences a different type of dilemma in the client, viz., the client's in India, by and large, show strong resistance to ventilate their very personal matters, viz., matter related to personal habits, sex-related matters, and so on to the counsellor, even though they prefer the counsellor to be directive in approach. Here, the counsellors direct approach fails; application of direct method to elicit such information gives a negative feeling to the counselee about the counsellor. Such clients may even misinterpret the counsellor, stating that the counsellor has brought to him/her some 'nasty' thoughts, which he/she dislikes. The counsellor, however, strongly believes that in such cases sexual guilt, inhibitions, perceived immoral/unethical interactions, etc. are the root cases of the given client's present problems.

(vii) In psychoanalytical approach, sometimes clients cognitive orientation to facts of life does not fit him/her well with such interpretation; in some other cases even though the client understands interpretation, he may, (a) deny altogether the fact, and (b) the interpretation itself induces guilt and conflict (a process of self-realisation). and thus it becomes a time consuming process; finally making the client feel disappointed).

In sum, the counsellors' dilemma in Indian set-up are two faceted :

(a) at certain stage of the counselling when the counsellor expects the client to take the counsellor in confidence and to disclose all required information, the client doesn't (resistance?); and

(b) at certain other stage of counselling when the counsellor desires that let the client be self-dependent and comply with non-directive approach, the client expects the contrary (insecurity?).

It is not necessary that either resistance or insecurity only will cause hindrance in the process of counselling; an admixture of similar qualities of client's personality may also delay the process. Such resistance at one stage and insecurity (ultimately both indicates unresolved conflicts leading to insecurity), at the other, are culturally determined.

Dilemma 3 : To reframe or refrain or retain some cultural phenomena : India is passing through a very significant phase of transition with regard to implementation of traditional values and norms of this culture by the younger generation. Though problems arising out of generation gap is a company phenomenon all over the world, India has been passing through a very acute phase of such problems. Western culture has moulded the life style of a significant section of our population, namely, the young and the adolescents. This has resulted in identity crises in the youth; behavioural manifestations of which are irritation and unrest in them. They are neither fully acculturated in the Western style, nor are they admirers of India's old traditional norms. This has caused lots of confusion in them and they are becoming increasingly resentful to authority figures. This causes lots of emotional problems in their parents too, particularly those who resist refraining from Indian traditional values and customs. Youngsters coming for counselling exhibit that their problems appear to be twofold :

(i) On the one hand, they have been totally dependent on their parents for their daily life activities; parents' direct involvements in their life activities has never been considered by them as interference. This, in turn, has encouraged parents to be more and more controlling; this thus jeoparadises the youngster's responsibility taking behaviour altogether;

(ii) on the other hand, for their very personal matters, viz., selection of friends, particularly that of the opposite sex, and even for the selection of life partners, they want to exercise their full freedom without any imminence of this change of behaviour (pertaining to this segment of their lives) to their parents. Consequently, they developed guilt; sometimes they suffer a lot emotionally because of their immature decision, and, on the other, parents/family members start showing high resistance to accept such independent decision of their wards.

(iii) Parents/family members sometimes create confusion in their offsprings because of their inconsistent behaviour in rewarding them.

(iv) Some of the parents, in spite of showing strong resistance to accept any deviation for their past, traditional family values and norms, simultaneously carve for behaviour patterns which are consonant with the present societal values.

The counsellor, in such circumstances, must have expertise to find an appropriate balance to help the young and their seniors. Because, in Indian set-up, even to solve the problems of the youth, parents/family members require to be consulted as because decision making is a collective endeavour. Once again, the counsellor is in a dilemma because he/she should not impose his/her values on either of the parties—the youth or the old—even if the counsellor realises that one of these parties may be correct, because in that case the other party usually misinterprets the counsellor's action as partiality in judgement. In that case the party who feels that the counsellor has shown partiality to the other party refrains from continuing further sessions, which is detrimental to both the parties.

As mentioned earlier, generally in Indian culture, a very low premium is given to the youngsters by the society for free mixing with the persons of the opposite sex. As a result women participating in higher education, and occupation become victims of family resentment in many ways in some circumstances. Such attitudinal differences between the old and the young is typical in India even with regard to the mode of selection of the life partners, viz., love marriage (preferred by the youngsters) versus arranged marriage (choice of the old generation). Of late, considering the outcome of marriage (be it love or arranged), and the Indian traditional cultural expectation, it becomes really difficult to provide judgement readily as to which type is preferred or acceptable for a given couple and their family members either.

Also, role conflict in women, namely, home role and occupational role is causing lots of adjustment problems in the youth and the old. Traditional expectation of the old generation may not necessarily go hand in hand with those of the young women. The counsellor, once again, has to balance between the two—remaining impartial to the clients. The problems faced with women of rural areas are quite different. Number of rural women who come forward for counselling is also very meagre.

These are some of the bidimensional issues peculiar to Indian culture. The counsellor has to widen his/her field of work to obtain balance between the traditionalism versus modernism, so that mental health of both the groups can be sustained adequately.

Dilemma 4 : Please refer to the vignettes of the youth cases mentioned earlier where initially though it appears that the youths are suitable for marital counselling, depth information revealed subsequently through interview (in some cases through psychometric tests required) possess questions—whether marital counselling to start with, would really help them to have long standing intevention outcome. Secondly, in come cases developmental counselling would be required, whilst for some others cognitive restructuring, and still for some others psychoanalytical approach. Thirdly, it is clear from the case vignettes that though both the partners while presenting their recent problems, talk of almost similar complains, their life experiences show different orientation. At this juncture the couple appear to be more different than they are similar. Unlike the couples where one of the partners volunteer, and the other resists to receive counselling services, when both the partners volunteer, their approach initially though appears to be very positive (motivational aspect), and unidimensional, later, on several occasions, their ultimate goal to come to a counsellor is found to be bidimensional in nature. In case vignette I, for instance, the would-be couple came together for counselling but their ulterior motive was bidirectional. That is, one of them was rigid enough to break the relation for ever, whilst the other was equally rigid to continue the relationship for ever (even now in India it prevails that once married to some one means—marriage would last for whole life). Thus, the mental rigidity that prevailed in the said couple was bidirectional. The girl showed positive rigid access for—whilst the boy showed rigidity to recede from—marriage. This causes dilemma in selecting methods of counselling. For example, whether client centred approach would be suitable here? In most of the cases, individual counselling separately for both the partners is required for long time with a view to prepare them for joint counselling. Sometimes clients raise questions as to why the counsellor is not discussing their problems jointly; likewise, time factor involved in individual counselling followed by joint sessions require explanation to the clients. If client does not want to compromise with time (because fails to foresee the outcome) they prefer to switch over to some other counsellor.

Dilemma 5 : Whether or not a counsellor can be decisively expressive in certain circumstances?

In the case vignette II above, the husband appeared twice, but reluctantly, perhaps to show his cooperation to his wife in this regard, though his indifferent attitude expressed during interview, and to the wife's problems in relation to his mother, gave a clear idea that he won't be perturbed even if his marriage breaks. The wife, too was totally disgusted with her husband's attitude, but with a faint ray of hope, as a last resort, came for counselling, just on a trial basis thinking if at all reconciliation would be possible. Here, the counsellor is to help the husband realise his inadequacies in context of exerting his role as a husband, particularly in taking steps to overcome his mother's interference in his and his wife's personal matters; but this is possible provided the husband would agree to attend the sessions. There may be several reasons for the husband showing resistance to attend the counselling sessions, and also for his indifferent attitude to retain his marital relation with his wife. The wife did not want to break the marriage provided the husband would cooperate in solving the stated problems.

In such circumstances, the counsellor normally is posited with certain questions which cause dilemma in him/her. For instance, the case under reference—here the wife raised two important queries to the counsellor—

(a) "Doctor do you think I can go for a second marriage"? Considering Indian culture, it is really a critical question to answer in yes/no fashion, and more so, if the counsellor has conducted counselling sessions in client-centred approach. The reasons why the client (wife) had asked this questions—(i) she has expressed insecurity and uncertainty about the possibility of her getting 2nd marriage on the ground of stigma which prevails in Indian society; (ii) she was found highly apprehensive about the 2nd husband's personality characteristics, and thus indecisive against whether to remarry. She has lost all confidence at this stage whether desired mental matching will be possible with the so-called prospective groom. Even if a counsellor, in certain cases, feels that divorce would be a right decision, in Indian cultural perspective, can a counsellor encourage divorce? Counsellor's duty is to see that a marriage lasts happily through reconciliation.

(b) Secondly, if the counsellor, remaining non-commital, suggests the wife (in this case), "Well if you can motivate your husband to come for counselling, then both of you could receive help for reconciliation".

The client : "See, I don't think my husband will come for counselling; however, if I can motivate him, how long it will take to reconcile the matter"?

The counsellor : "I cannot spell out exact time and number of sessions to be required. It all depends upon you as to how quickly you learn to modify your thoughts, feelings, expectations, and actions" (counsellor non-commital).

The Client : "Doctor, supposing it takes long time, say years together, if at all my husband modifies his behaviour, by the time, I would be 30+; so long I don't find certainty about my husband's future behaviour, I would have to postpone, though reluctantly, my motherhood. Supposing he agrees to reconcile and to have a child, I will be so late to start my life, to bring up my children (if at all I can conceive and so on). That's what I am worried about."

The counsellor : (To remain non-commital). Well, you are to adjust accordingly.

At this stage the dilemma in the counsellor—If, in such complicated cases, where clients have deep-rooted personality problems, viz., extreme dependency onto the mother, and related other inadequacies, for the husband, obviously phychoanalytical approach would be required. The counsellor realises very well that the whole process will take long time, particularly when—

(i) the husband has shown strong resistance so far to receive such services. Also, what all the wife so far stated about her future life plan is very correct;

(ii) wife's insecurity about 2nd husband's personality etc., if at all she goes for a second marriage (wife is apprehensive if that too ends in a divorce);

(iii) Indian scenario, discourages repeated divorce and marriage, and problems becomes acute when the client is very sensitive about the societal norm.

Considering (i), (ii) and (iii), can a counsellor advice the client to go for remarriage? What would be the socio-legal consequences onto the counsellor? Would the counsellor be mentally ready to bear adverse consequences?

Dilemma 6 : When clients' perception of a problem and motivation to ameliorate the same are not unidirectional

In case vignette I above, the would-be couple came for counselling with a common problem, i.e., maladjustment in them now itself at the premarital stage (same perception of the problem by both); both apprehensive whether marital life will be happy (both apprehensive of future adjustment). But to ameliorate the problem the male partner does not want this girl while the female partner is stubborn to see that marriage takes place between them only (means employed to ameliorate the problem—bi-directional).

In case vignette III above, the couple's perception of the problem is same, i.e., marital disharmony. But motivation to ameliorate the problem is bi-directional—whether the husband not willing to come for counselling; the husband shows vacillation in decision, e.g., sometimes thinks that this marriage can last (purchased flat to stay separately) and sometimes rigid to break the marriage (warned his wife to go for separation). The wife, though willing to come for counselling, showed ambivalence in the sense that sometimes expressed her impatience in settling her life, whilst, on the other, resisted husband's threat of divorce ((telling the husband "when we agreed to marry, marriage is not to break, so you are to see that our relationship goes well with happiness").

In the above examples, both the males have inadequacy, and needs to escape, whereas both the females have need to possess. With regard to both the males their tendency to escape is also encouraged by their parents. With regard to both the females their tendency to possess is also encouraged by their parents, particularly by their respective fathers. In one of these 2 cases, the father of the girl reported that it is due to her mother's inspiration that the girl was so stubborn (which was disliked by the father of the girl throughout); such a situation (triangular in nature) required parents' counselling for both the parties separately. Parents were unwilling to come for it. As a result, counselling of the parents, and also group counselling for both the parents and the clients together can't be held. How can the counsellor do justice to the clients (in the above example, particularly when both the female partners who expect that the counsellor can solve their problems) under such circumstances?

Dilemma 7 : When amelioration of the clients' problem begets several other related problems into the family members of the clients and vice-versa

The case vignettes V and VI of the youths, mentioned above, are typical of Indian scenario with regard to the marriage of sons/daughters. Both the clients are willing to go for engagement according to their own choice, but parents strongly object. Naturally question arises : who requires counselling? The answer is not that stgraight forward, if the counsellor is aware of Indian culture. Though in both the cases, the clients have come forward, interestingly, while coming for counselling sessions they (the clients) were accompanied by their parents. One might assume taking it as a positive gesture that both the clients and their parents came together, so counselling of the clients and parents would be easier. But gradual probe into the matter brings a negative impression. Because separate interview with the clients and their parents bring onto the surface the fact that the very purpose of coming for counselling is different for the clients than that of their parents. Thus, incongruity prevails in the family regarding selection of the son's/daughter's life partner. Parents, on the one hand, want to maintain cultural tradition in the sense of exercising their authority in deciding over such matter. The sons/daughters, on the other, though want to exercise their individuality, cannot exert themselves because of their—(i) dependency on the parents, (ii) to fulfil their moral and social obligations to their parents. Because, if the marriage takes place without the consent of the respective parents, parents might not allow them to maintain any relation with them, in that case sons/daughters will develop guilt feeling as they will fail to perform their duties to their respective parents. To avoid such guilt, in such cases, sons/daughters expect that their personal choice be consented by their parents. Many a times such expectations do not get fulfilled. In such circumstances, generally, newly married couple faces a sort of humiliation by the society in the sense that they have failed to perform their duties to their respective parents—particularly at this age of the parents when they really need mental and physical support from their sons/daughters in many respects; absence of which may even cause serious emotional problems and social humiliation to the parents. Thus many of our youths are susceptible to experience guilt which is bidimensional in nature : one from the point of view of their parents (failure to perform duties up to the parents' expectation) and the other from the point of view of their failure to retain words and kinship. They become mostly the victims of a strong dilemma—whether to refrain from the former duty or to maintain the latter (commitments). Strictly speaking, the former is considered no less a commitment than the latter in Indian interpersonal interactional scenario.

Such a scenario of interaction has many positive as well as negative aspects, which have been discussed in detail before in this book and need not be repeated here.

In separate interview the parents expressed their desire stating "Dr., please help us; please see that he/she does not get married to his/her partner; he/she can't foresee that such marriage will not last long". The clients, on the contrary, stated, "Dr., please convince my parents; if I don't marry this proposed partner, I won't marry for the whole life. Moreover, I have committed, if I retreat now, the partner may even commit suicide. How can I go to office or college if such a litigation arises against me, and also you know doctor..."

One might think, and,of course, it is very easy to think that counselling be done separately for the clients and the parents and to make a common platform based on give-and-take policy. In actuality, in India scenario, its not that easy a job for the counsellor, particularly if we consider the consequences—both legal and social—which take place in our culture sometimes in extreme form.

As a simile it may be stated that when a hypertensive mother punishes her child, the child eagerly looks towards his father for rescue; the child, as if, prays to his father for help, which if unobtained the child feels like his mother's prey; if father resists mother, the mother feels highly perturbed and highstrung; if father does not rescue the child, the child becomes highly frustrated. Such a dilemma of a family often occurs to a clincial counsellor in Indian set-up when counselling.

Dilemma 8 : Dilemma between maintaining offence and providing defence

When the client trusts the genuineness of the counsellor and understands his empathetic sharing of the client's problems, that creates a ground for the client to unveil all his guilt and shame to the counsellor with a view to seek his/her advice to overcome his conflicts. Such catharisis is very helpful in counselling outcome but creates dilemma on the part of the counsellor. For example,

Client : Dr., I have another very important issue to discuss with you which has been haunting me especially since our last session's discussion. Can I tell you that?

Counsellor : Yes, if you so desire.

Client : I had a very bad incident in my life when I was appearing for H.S. exam. That very incident has made a scar in my life and, I think, that is the cause of my obtaining unexpectedly bad scores in the Board Examination (compared to my previous examinations where throughout I was a topper).

Counsellor : Really, an incident which you think has a causal impact on your obtaining low score in the exam?

Client : Yes. I had a sexual interaction (not intercourse) with my distant relative, which later others come to know and they have accused me; even the girl blamed me later, though a number of times she gave me consent for the same.

Counsellor : Let's discuss how, in general, you think, such an event can cause poor results in examinations (matter was discussed in client-centred approach). In subsequent sessions, the client, in context of his own result, understood that it is a cultural norm which has caused guilt in him and self-imposed punishment was there, as he said at this stage "I perhaps, wanted a bad score in the Board examination to make my face down to the others" (need for self-punishment expressed).

Client : I would like to know from you whether I can disclose this to my fiancée, whom I would like to marry after a couple of years? I have developed the relation after that bad incident; I know that my fiancée is very honest and considers me to be equally honest. I am in a dilemma that— "if I don't unveil this to her, I feel I am deceiving her, on the other hand, I am afraid, she might discontinue this affair (which would be unbearable to me), if I disclose this to her." Again, "I am afraid that she might commit suicide (sense of rejection) thinking that I like someone else more than her". If the latter, "I may have to be victimised socially and legally, and also personally and morally".

This is a dilemma to counsellor as well particularly in Indian culture, where sex before marriage is not accepted, as the concept of divorce has not yet been easily accepted by the society. Break in affairs is usually taken with a sense of rejection by the youngsters. One might suggest that it would be much easier to solve the problem if both the partners would have joined for counselling. But, once again, in Indian culture, the other partner does not normally agree to come for joint counselling excepting the one who takes initiative to receive such assistance. He male partner came for counselling focussing his problems of lack of concentration in studies and consequent unexpected results in the Board Examination (though underlined factor was different as revealed later). Such an excuse might be accepted by his girl-friend (if at all he discloses this information to her that he has been receiving help from a counsellor). But one doesn't dare to disclose his other problem (sex-related) to his fiancée to get her motivated to come for counselling, with the apprehension that affair may break. Of course, if the partners had had such a deep understanding with each other that even if he discloses this later to his girl friend even then the relation wouldn't break. In that case, thy may not require counselling, for such matter.

In sum, when a client expresses such perceived offences, it is for the counsellor to decide whether and when to break such perseverance (to avoid possible break-down); or to equip him with defences to maintain his psychological well-being.

Dilemma 9 : Focus of attention : The client or the stated problem(s)

A girl, 25 yrs, graduate, employed, married for last 18 months, affair with her present husband lasted for about 6 months. Since marriage disharmony evident between them to the extent that question of divorce has been raised by the family members of the husband. The wife came for counselling. She appeared to be very possessive and aggressive; associated complaints of lack of concentration, sleep disturbance, easy irritability, were reported. The mother of the client described the client as very stubborn and egoistic throughout. The client described her husband as meek, unassertive, mother dependent and easily suggestive by parents. The husband has never been available during the counselling sessions. In one of the sessions, the client asked a direct question to the counsellor "Would you advice me to go for divorce, doctor, though I personally can't bear to designate myself as a 'divorcee', if situation demands so," As already mentioned, a counsellor cannot give a directive to go for divorce on medico-legal grounds, unless otherwise reported (e.g., medically provided unfit, etc.). Nothing like the latter was reported in this case.

Whether to focus on the client or on the problems reported during counselling? For the beginners particularly, though the temptation is to focus on the problems and to solve it immediately, sometimes to focus on the client—rather onto the problem—gives longterm benefit. However, it depends upon the orientation of the counsellor. The client-centred and psychoanalytical orientation prefer to focus on the client first, whereas behaviourists would prefer to focus on the problems first. It depends however, upon the counsellors' ability to judge (considering the merit of the case) whether the client or the problem be focussed initially.

For the above case, it was evident that the wife required counselling largely from the point of view of her personality. She expressed a dilemma—to go for divorce (when she experiences severe distress) and to avoid the designation of a divorcee. If, as in one-way traffic, the counsellor tries to hold the client to modify her orientation towards marriage, her attitude, and so on, she required enduring patience to get relief from her presenting distress. If she could really change her attitude, etc. the present marriage may not break. But certain irrationalities, inadequacies of the husband reported by her (if true), unless modified, how long the client (wife) can have this attitude to forgive and forget? Had she been having that type of attitude she would not have to come for counselling at all. If, however, she can change her attitude, orientation etc, towards marriage and life interaction, she might save herself from future breaking-off in marriage if she gets divorce in this case and remarries (second marriage).

So, to save the client from the presenting distress, if she is advised to see that the present marriage lasts at least for a few months more, then she requires at least a minimum emotional support from her present husband. But her present husband is not at all cooperative to attend counselling sessions, neither individually, nor jointly.

As reported by the wife the husband also seems to have some personality problems which require psychological probing. If the client really wants to avoid others calling her a 'divorcee', she should have that lavel of patience that she could bear everything happening in the family. But she is not like that; which also may not necessarily be true for many others.

Practically she can't accept the term 'divorcee' but in actuality she is fed up with the present husband's attitude and behaviour towards her. To save the client from her present problems, i.e., approach-avoidance conflict regarding retaining marital relationship with the present husband, should the counsellor focus on the present problem, or her basic personality disposition?

Incidents of marital disharmony could be reduced significantly provided the would-be couple could come forward for pre-marital counselling. There too, attitudinal differences of the male and the female cause a great hindrance. In India, many are not aware of the availability of such services, those who are aware, show strong resistance to receive such services as because—

(i) they think that the counselling is required for mentally ill persons;

(ii) they are apprehensive that during the process of counselling many hidden complexes of them would come to the surface and ultimately marriage may not take place (rigidly wants to move by the influence of infatuation, without considering long term consequencies); this of course is an indication of their immaturity;

(iii) that they require counselling—if such information gets divulged to the society, their affair will never turnout into reality—they are apprehensive of it.

Chapter 16

COUNSELLING: INDIGENOUS MODEL

Bankground Information

There is a rapid socio-cultural transformation in Indian culture. It is passing through a significant phase of transition in implementing its traditional values and norms in daily life interaction. Western culture has moulded the life style of a significant section of our population, particularly the younger generation. Our younger generation are neither following the old values totally, nor have they been acculturated with the Western values fully. This has caused lots of confusion in them, so much so that several of the Indian values and norms are being severally questioned by them. Psychologically, they are experiencing crises in terms of their identity. As a result, the youth are becoming increasingly resentful to authority, particularly those who are the followers of traditional, conservative values and norms. The behavioural manifestations of such resentment are causing irritation and unrest in them.

Leaving aside the adolescents and the younger section, some people, even in their middle adulthood, though show a tendency to resist separation from the old norms and traditions, simultaneously carve for things which are not in consonance with past values. Such incongruities in them causes lot of confusions in others—particularly those who interact with them directly. Such intraindividual and interindividual value clash causes problems of adjustment in both the young and in the old.

The issue of gender discrimination is another burning problem in this culture, even though the magnitude of the problem is waning recently. Largely, in the urban and semi-urban set-up, women are not debarred from educational and occupational facilities in life. But in rural areas, particularly in remote villages, women are victims of such issue; they are considered the weaker gender, and are deprived of life facilities enjoyed by the males. The problems which women of the rural set-up experience are different in nature compared to those of the women of the urban areas. Various reasons for this are—largely the women of the rural areas are housewives, are less educated, may even be illiterate. This could be used as a pointer to the need arrange awareness programmes for them so that necessary counselling services can be catered.

Gender discrimination seems to prevail even today in Indian society in connection with role-expectation. Though recently both gender discrimination and role expectation have changed its trend to a certain extent, even then women—irrespective of their education, occupation and area of habitation—seem to have some additional roles to play in everyday life adjustment compared to their male counterparts. Such variations in the nature and degree of role expectations create confusions, conflicts, and even crises in adjustment many a times, particularly in the seniors. This, once again, reflects incongruity in our expectation. Such incongruity is between traditionalism versus modernism in implementation of our social values and norms, particularly for the women section. For example, women's double role—namely, home role and occupational role and corresponding expectations by the society—obviously bear counselling implications. At par with the modern trend, many families have accepted the occupational role of women, but many families, on the contrary, cannot forgive such employed women, if they fail to perform their home role adequately like housewives. Housewives, on the other hand, in some cases complain of inferiority and fear of dependence, when they are not allowed to go for service, by their in-laws, in spite of having adequate qualifications required. These issues are to be dealt with adequately in context of our culture.

Attitudinal differences prevail mostly between the older generation (including some middle aged group) and some modern people, regarding the sphere of interaction of our youth, particularly with the persons of the opposite sex. Such restricted interaction does debar many of our women from taking part in higher education and occupation. Many a times, employed women, and women who intend to pursue higher education, become victims of family unrest. This problem becomes more acute when married women fail to receive support from their respective husbands in favour of continuing education or occupation. Counsellor has to widen his/her field of work to consider such problems which are unique to India.

Attitudinal differences between the old and the young also result in family disharmony, particularly when youngsters favour love marriages, as against that of negotiated marriage; mostly the latter is accepted and approved by the seniors. Under such circumstances, youngsters come to the counsellor with an intention to seek help in the sense that if the counsellor could convince their parents to accept the 'affair'. The parents, on the contrary, seek help from the counsellor as if the counsellor would be able to convince the youngsters to break the 'affair'. Whether love marriage is more successful than negotiated one, in Indian culture, is a separate issue and its detailing is beyond the scope of this book. From the above dichotomous issue it is clear that the main concern of counselling in such cases turns out to be totally different from its expected goal. That is, whether the match would be a suitable one for future life happiness becomes insignificant; on the contrary, the issue of right and wrong, regarding the mode of selection of the partners, as per social norms, becomes more significant to the counsellor. Counsellor's duty is not to pass on verdict as to who is right and who is wrong, but to make the would be couple realise whether marriage is likely to end in success. Such a bidimensional issue has to be tackled by the counsellor considering our old values and traditions on the one hand, and attitudinal differences between the youths and their seniors, on the other.

Incidence of marital disharmony could be reduced significantly provided the youths would come forward for pre-marital counselling. Unfortunately, in India, many youths even today are not aware of the benefit of such services. Those who are aware too show strong resistance to receive such services, probably because (a) a significant section of such youths think that counselling is for mentally ill persons; (b) some of them are afraid that during counselling some of their psychological shorticomings might come in the forefront and, consequently, their marriage may not take place (apprehension of separation), and (c) quite a few of them are apprehensive that from the counsellor, their parents and the other members of the family may come to know about their affair which will cause a great hindrance to materialisation of their affair into marriage. This of course, shows once again their ignorance about the role of a counsellor. The counsellor's duty is not to divulge private information publicly. Attitudinal differences between the senior and junior sections of our population is causing such a problem in our culture.

The main focus of counselling, though in general is to help the client feel competent in independent decision-making, in India, this issue possesses a significant problem. This problem, in turn, causes dilemma both in the client as well as in the counsellor. From the client's point of view—by and large, our adolescents and youths show incongruity—their need to depend on their seniors versus tendency to defy seniors. Mostly tendency to defy develops when they feel frustrated owing to their inability to fulfil their need to depend. As mentioned earlier in this book, Indian child-rearing practices and family interactions style mostly do not encourage autonomy, independence and ability to execute decisions promptly and individually; youngsters are expected to consult family seniors even for petty matters. To a certain extent decisions are culturally determined. In the West, on the contrary, these are considered negative attributes of personality. Therefore, in Indian model of counselling, one has to be careful whether approach like that of the Roger's client centred would really help, at least in the initial sessions of the counselling, where the clients, on an average, would expect from the counsellor to guide him/her through direct approach. Of course it does not mean that whatever the client wants the counsellor has to comply with, but initial non-directive approach may not encourage many of our clients to continue sessions, as because they want immediate resolution of their problems in forms of direct command from the counsellor.

Herein develops some dilemma in the counsellor : The counsellors' dilemmas have different angles—(a) the counsellor knows very well that such dependency of the client has to be modified, still then, he/she can't initiate counselling sessions in the desired direction; (b) the counsellor aims to the help the client learn how to overcome such dependency, still, to comply with the client, at least to initiate intervention sessions, the counsellor might have to remain non-committal at least for a short span regarding such undesired behaviour of the client, which, in turn, is likely to hamper the time-budget of the counsellor to reach the stage of termination; (c) counselling in real sense of the term does not allow the counsellor to impos his/her thoughts, ideas, and values upon the client, even then the counsellor may have to initiate sessions in a direction which is different from that of his/her own choice, just to save the client from further damage in terms of the client's insecurity—disappointments, and even from life threat—depending upon the crises the client reports.

The counsellors' dilemma becomes more complicated when he/she finds incongruity amongst our clients in executing their needs (dependence/independence). Contrary to dependency, noted in majority of our clients, a good number of adolescents and youths show resistance for quite sometimes to take the counsellor in confidence while revealing their very core personal issues, namely, sexual matters. They show lots of inhibitions to verbalise their inner feelings and guilt etc., even though they are totally perturbed with such issues. Once again, the counsellor understands very well the roots of the client's problems, but can't impose upon his/her thoughts on to the clients, If the counsellor employs psychoanalytical approach, the clients may not necessarily understand the implications of such interpretation many a times, and a good number of clients deny altogether such implications, even though they are aware of such events/experiences in their life. Client-centred approach too may not be applicable in such cases, may be because they don't fulfil the criteria for the same.

In sum, counsellors' dilemma in Indian set-up is two-faceted : (i) at a certain stage of the counselling when the counsellor expects the client to take him/her into confidence, the client doesn't (resistance?), (ii) while at certain other stage of counselling, the counsellor desires that the client be self-dependent, the client expects the contrary (insecurity?). Such resistance at one stage and insecurity on the other are culturally determined, and are to be dealt with adequately during counselling.

Need for indigenisation of counselling/psychotherapy has been felt long back (Sinha and Holtzman, 1984) and, accordingly, attempts have already been made for it (e.g., Neki, 1973, 1976). A comprehensive review on this matter is available (Rangaswami, 1996). Andrew, Dias-Sexena and Patel (2000) described the rationale, development, and piloting of counselling intervention for general/common mental discorders seen in India.

It is not uncommon to a clinician that many of the conflicts noted in the clients are reflective of those experienced by the clients during the process of development, no matter which culture the client belongs to. Child rearing practices, family interactions, peer and social group influence, protective factors and social supports available, socio-cultural values etc. are important determinants for the development of psychopathology. Since process of socialisation has a large and significant impact onto the development of behavioural problems in the clients, a counsellor in Indian set-up has to have a model which is suitable to our culture—both for probing into and understanding the problem; and also in implementation of its intervention strategy. The problems reported by the clients are long established patterns of behaviour, exhibited as early as childhood or adolescence; but mostly such problems remain unnoticed and even uncared for at the beginning. Behaviours such as aggressive actions, passive aggressiveness, attention seeking, dependency etc. are long established patterns of an individual and cannot be remedied on the spot as the clients expect. The counsellor has to know first the process of socialisation of the client through which such undesired behaviour becomes part of a person's behavioural repertoire. Many Indian researchers (Nandy, 1976; Kakar, 1976; Hoch, 1990) reported that separation and individuation of the self does not take place in the Indian children at the rate and intensity expected in the West. This seems to promote prolonged infancy (Kakar, 1976) and foster dependency in Indian children.

Model

A model consists of a set of assumptions about a system (Maher, 1970). Model has certain characteristics. A detailed discussion of these would b beyond the scope of this chapter. However, for the present purpose, we shall consider the assumption of a model as the properties of it. A model would help in understanding psychopathology.

Model 1 : Conflict on the Issue of Dependence-Independence

The following is an attempt to formulate some tentative models to understand psychopathology in context to our culture. One such model is to deal with conflicts. The most commonly noted conflict in our clients, particularly in the adolescents and youths, is the issue of dependence-independence. Their need to depend is not compatible with (a) their age related maturity in some cases, and (b) with the expectation of the society from them, in some other cases. The former, though such individuals are matured by age and have accomplished certain status and position in the society, fail to exert themselves accordingly due to excessive dependency. They, in fact, are not able to enjoy their achievements and accomplishment in the real sense of the term. In the latter, though they have developed adequate age-related maturity, self-reliance and self-image, fail to satisfy the society (their demands is to be dependent) by sharing and depending upon them in decision-making. In the former, these individuals are mostly found to be uncertain and insecure; this causes incongruence in their orientation too, in respect of their perception of a phenomenon or event and in deciding upon their future action strategy. Some very commonly reported incongurities are overlapping between need to depend versus need for autonomy; need to depend versus fear of being overpowered. In the latter, their self-image, self-reliance, self-confidence do not adhere to the social expectation to comply with the social norms in decision-making. Unlike the former, the latter individuals do not prefer to succumb to others' authority. Thus the latter group experiences incongruity in mastering self and mastering one's environment satisfactorily. Incongruity between the perception of the self and that of the reality causes deep-rooted personal distress in such individuals. Incongruence makes these clients prone to feel threatened by realistic feedback about them from others.

Our model involves termendous aid in the development of self-esteem in the clients. This is to prove one's adequacy in standing alone, deciding alone, acting alone, and finally to perceive that he/she can accomplish alone. Clients mostly appear inept and ineffective in this regard. They even fail to take adequate efforts which would be self-rewarding. This is because they mostly lack perseverance to achieve as they have been reinforced during the past to get 'readymade achievements', without exercising perseverance. As a result, they can neither execute their plans to get reward, nor can wait for deferred reward.

In such cases, our counselling strategy may require relatively longer tenure compared to the frequently quoted classical techniques depicted in the literature of the other culture. Longer duration, because our clients, even in the counselling sessions, appear to be rigid in disclosing information out of social inhibition. Therefore, they show resistance to consent to any modifications of their cognitive structure, which deems suitable for them by the counsellor. This is no exception with regard to the client-centred approach too. After a few sessions of discussion, when a given client can realise the need for modification, in general, they take time again to execute the same. So, our model's prime focus is to deal with both the client's inhibitions (to disclosure of information) and resistance (to implement something new). Simultaneously, a moot question which requires answering at this stage is : why resistance? As mentioned earlier, resistance in counselling session is not a unique phenomenon. But in this culture, of all the other factors, one such is fear of failure in implementing, and in consequence fear of losing the original object of dependency. Such a fear once again reflects lack of self-confidence of the client(s), to change over from the old/traditional (though incorrect) to that of a new (uncertain) one. The clients with history of high reinforcement from need like dependency find it quite difficult to change.

At this state the very purpose of counselling might pose a question to both the counsellor and the counselee. Because the client seems to possess and remove the same thought/action pattern he desires to modify through counselling. The counsellor must not be disappointed. Such a dilemma in the client, in essence, should provide a positive cue to the counsellor that incongruities present in the client's thoughts are apparent to him, and the counsellor's task here is to see that the client remains motivated to continue sessions, so that the counsellor can help him/her to gain ultimately through such intervention. This, thus, is a significant pointer to the counsellor that the counselling process is likely to come to an end successfully.

Subsequent sessions are to be devoted to probing and make the client understand the purpose of holding contradictory desires simultaneously. For example, a 26 yr male, B.E., unmarried, employed, reported for stammering cure. He has had history of stammering since his 6th standard at school. He experiences severe stammering, though occasional, while meeting significant persons (like office boss) in his life. In initial few sessions he appeared highly defensive; though occasionally revealed some significant contradictions in his desires with reluctance. To name some such most significant contradictions—strong mother dependency versus need to excel as an employee (he fails), need to execute the role of an assertive husband, but expressed unwillingness to marry; wants to go abroad but lacks confidence regarding self-help in absence of mother; wants to earn name but at the same time possesses desire to humiliate himself. Cognitive therapeutic mode in client-centred approach revealed after 8th session that (i) he fails in asserting himself (when necessary) in his office environment, feels like having mother's support there too; (ii) unwilling to get married with an apprehension of getting detached from mother's support; (iii) he has lots of guilt related to sex, which impinges upon a strong sense of self-punishment; (iv) stammering has been serving double purpose (gain?) in him—on the one hand he succeeds in getting self-humiliation (when he stammers in front of others), and, on the other, it is a defense to gain sympathy and attention of others, particularly in work place, and social meets (as if this is the reason he can't excel—otherwise he is competent).

Thus question arises, does the client really want to get rid of his problem since he has some psychological gain (need satisfaction) out of this? Compared to the negative consequences, positive consequences of stammering appear more to him. However, such incongruities in thought once again are significant cues to the counsellor that the client has arrived at a state of self-understanding, though vacillates occasionally, showing resistance to implement the strategies he logically approves through counselling.

Our model, even to remove a physical complaint, viz., stammering, in this case, requires the client's mothers' involvement in counselling set-up. Incidentally, the client being the only son, the mother was found very possessive; in fact she took more time to modify her decisions and action patterns than the time taken by the client himself. Family structure revealed a nuclear family where the father of the client remains passive, which is again unlike the traditional Indian culture. Usually father becomes the controlling authority of the whole family (particularly for the external affairs) and the mother becomes the controlling authority (particularly for the internal affairs) in context of child-rearing issues, the excess of which encourages mother-dependence. To modify the client's mother's action pattern, here, for the given client his father's intervention was also required. So far as the major symptom is concerned (here stammering), one might think of behaviour therapy as the method of choice. But in this case, cognitive restructuring technique helped not only the client but his parents too to attain a desired state of behaviour. Incidentally, mention be made here that the client has been exposed to other traditional methods of treatment prior to reporting to this counsellor, but all in vain. This shows that culture bound modification is required in applying a technique for a given client, instead of grouping certain symptoms with some particular type of counselling techniques available in the classical text.

Model 2 : On Role Playing

The way men and women portray themselves is largely determined by a given culture (Bishop, 1992). Likewise, men and women, in any society, are influenced in determining their gender role, viz. to adopt the social mores, beliefs, attitudes and behaviour throughout their life. It is the 'scripting or training of children by parents, caregivers and others regarding behaviour, attitudes and expectations which are considered appropriate to the child's gender in the society or culture' (Bleier, 1991, p. 66). Thus role playing varies over culture.

By and large, in Indian society, during childhood upbringing, very high premium is always given to those behavioural action patterns which are described as modest, sober, and submissive, hardly any assertiveness is encouraged. The whole purpose behind such encouragement is to see that our children, i.e., tomorrow' adults, be accepted and approved by the society to its maximum, i.e., they be recognised as well behaved, good mannered and so on. Such reinforcement, depending upon its degree and frequency, at times make our adolescents incapable to exert themselves even if the situation arises. In such circumstances, contrary to their expectation, they are recognised by the society as inept, ineffective and, to its extreme, even inadequate in role playing. In this way, assertiveness is misinterpreted by them as aggressiveness. Since they don't learn to be assertive, finally the very essence of their behavioural characteristics, to be well 'mannered', well 'behaved' is also lost when, in certain situations, the latter is not entertained by the society.

Our youth, at a certain stage of their life, find themselves in utter confusion (exceptions are not ruled out). On the one hand, they fail to (in some circumstances, e.g., work place) meet-up with the expectation of others (lack of assertiveness), and, on the other, they can't accept others' imposition on them (resistance). The latter is interpreted by them as taking 'advantage' of them (feeling of being exploited). They develop resistance to such 'advantage'-taking attitude, but once again fails to express such resistant (to authority, e.g.), activity. Passive aggression develops in them. The whole spectrum develops out of their wrong interpretation of 'assertiveness' and 'aggressiveness'. These two may not necessarily overlap in real life. Assertiveness, in actuality, implies will to overt action, whilst aggressiveness includes hostility. Likewise, subsmissiveness must not mean to be meękly compliant as assertiveness must not mean to be aggressively dominating.

Advocates of aggressive communication, e.g., Alberti and Emmons (1995), suggest that submissiveness in extreme form leads to poor self-esteem, self-denial, emotional suppression and strained interpersonal relations. Aggressive communication, conversely, leads to guilt, alienalion and disharmony. Assertive behaviour, however. fosters high self-esteem, effective conflict management, and satisfactory interpersonal relations. Therefore, assertiveness and aggressiveness must not be bracketed.

One of the advantages of assertiveness is that it makes the individual ready to express his needs directly. It may not necessarily always ensure one to get his needs fulfilled readily, but, at times, does pave way to possibilities for future fulfilment. In our society non-assertiveness of the youth gets manifested in the following ways : (i) at the personal domain failure in academic achievement; (ii) in occupational domain fear of taking responsibility, though the person aspires social status in occupation; as a result they complain of depression on promotion. In the family interaction domain—fear of failure in adjustment with the parents, and with the wife in the marital sphere of life. In the broader social sphere of life—fear of failure to keep interaction with other and subsequent fear of criticisms by others. Such individuals also report frequent physical complaints, similar to that of hypertension, and hypocondriasis. All these problems are largely due to their strong dependency on others, and due to lack of self-confidence in decision-making in spite of they possessing very good academic record. For e.g., a male (26 yrs), employed in IT sector reported during counselling "Dr., I could have no problem in performing my duties at office with full responsibility, provided I could have got my father sitting by my side in my office..." He feels proud describing him 'modest' (which has made his self-esteem very poor) and 'sober' (which has made him meek and submissive) compared to his colleagues with whom he had been facing problems of adjustment (they are not sober as per the client). This illustration must not give an impression that the author is against modest behaviour. What is intended to mention here is that modesty, soberness are thus being misinterpreted sometimes by some of our youths. Another problem which we come across is extreme mother dependency, particularly for some males. This causes separation anxiety in them after marriage; they feel very insecured to enact the role of a competent husband. Such passivity is not encouraged by their wives, but their parents sometimes prefer their sons to be dependent on them and to follow their directions even after marriage. These youths are in a fix between two bi-directional role expectations, namely, passivity/dependency versus assertiveness.

In such instances, our counselling model does not fit in well with the classical marital counselling model applied in respect to the couples of other culture. Here individual counselling of the couple would be the method of choice initially; thereafter parental counselling followed by family counselling to maintain emotional equilibrium of both the parents and the married couple. Such individuals are usually hypertensive and, as such, they get involved in a sort of "civil war", described by Suinn (1975). "Civil War" is between "passive dependency" versus "aggressive assertiveness" (Suinn, 1975). These require dynamic interpretation and thus are time—taking.

Compared to an individual who is open and clearly hostile, it is difficult to interact with passive-aggressive individuals. The latter group is stubborn and resistant. During counselling session elements of controversies become prominent in them, as a result it takes long time to get their inner negativisim expressed during the session, though often these clients show a picture of superficial cooperation. This is reflected in their resistance to finish-up homework assigned to them, e.g., in a cognitive therapeutic paradigm. Such resistance becomes apparent repeatedly with some lame excuses, viz., forgetfulness. When they are placed in a behavioural orientation programme, they decline to participate; if participate, not whole-heartedly. For example, they want to misuse phone access or e-mail access of the counsellor prior to reporting for the assigned session to the counsellor's office and so on. During discussion sessions, they normally go on focussing on minute details of some incidents/events for clarifications, which is not required at this stage of intervention. They thus delay action continuously. This is because they have conflict between need to depend versus fear of being dominated. They want to compromise by being dependent through passivity, and avoiding domination through resistance. Unfortunately, such a compromise is not conductive to quick intervention outcome.

Model 3 : To deal with deep-rooted guilt of the clients

Cross-cultural differences in the mode of treatment of emotionally disturbed are clearly definable. Such differences are mainly due to differences in attitudes which can have significant impact onto the therapeutic endeavour. Levine (1972) long before hypothesized that such attitudinal differences are result of the 'physicians more general socio-political belief sructures about all social issues rather than being more narrowly related to their concepts of mental illness alone'. In our society, we face problems related to social issues and attitudinal differences in counselling sessions too, which are predominantly culturally determined family related issues mostly raised by our clients. Dispositions of guilt, as one such vital issue, is to be attributed to the rigid convictions which the society has planted in our children.

Many of our clients, irrespective of their age, sex, education, socio-economic status are found to be plagued by excessive guilt even on some petty matters. Clients with depression, OCD, hypohcondriasis, conversion hysteria, examination phobia, marital disharmony, and even those with stammering are some such examples. The clinical symptoms they represent do not apparently bear any relation to their experience of severe guilt. Further probe into the etiological aspects of the reported symptoms does reveal presence of significant level of guilt in them, and these are all based on our social values and norms. However, degree of guilt and phenomena related to it are diverse in nature. Let us examine some of the most commonly reported phenomena related to guilt. At the very personal sphere of life, guilt is mostly sexual in nature, viz., masturbatory guilt, being sexually seduced during adolescence. Similarly guilt in the youth related to incestual imagination (though no action really), nudity even when alone in bathroom or in a confinement, voyeurism, and, in some cases, heterosexual interaction etc. which cause lack of concentration, memory failure, examination phobia in adolescents, and hypochondriasis, hysterical symptom manifestation and the like in the young adults, which—in extreme form—causes fear of death. Such individuals possess a need to banish sexual thoughts, because sex is perceived by them as a lewd act; as the act is indecent and dirty, it is punishable. Similar guilt is also found to be present in some of the adults as well which gets manifested in the form of OCD and the like even at their late 40s. Counselling when aims to shake the clients' rigid cognitive orientation requires quite a few sessions in such cases.

Considering the age of the client, cognitive restructuring may be done on the one hand by providing the client with adequate knowledge about sex as an instinct and about normal functions of sex hormones in human organism, and, on the other, by providing the client knowledge about the psychodynamic interpretation behind such symptom manifestation; that is, how somatic complaints develop out of psychic conflicts. In the former, though the client understands thaf sex is a normal and universal phenomenon, still the client remains in confusion in the subsequent sessions stating that he/she fails to reconcile between logic and emotion. That is, logically though he/she understand normal physiological functions of sex, can't refrain himself/herself from the apprehension that his sexual thoughts and/or action will bring on some punishment (guilt induced). At this juncture, if the client is provided with adequate knowledge about the sources and functions of guilt, i.e., how guilt functions as a cultural ingredient, as a last resort, the client appears to seek assurance from the counsellor whether he/she will be forgiven by the family, in particular, and the society, in general. Likewise, in the adult cases, if the source of guilt is found to be wife, for example, ultimately the husband, after a few sessions, needs assurance from wife and vice versa, because, as a last resort, our clients, irrespective of their age, wants to verify whether he/she has been forgiven by the source (object) of guilt feelings. Thus, the client even at this stage of counselling seems to depend on the mercy of others' acceptance and approval. Such a situation demands inclusion of the respective parents/guardians of the client(s) in the counselling sessions. There too, we come across a problem. Some of the clients easily agree to sit with their parents jointly in the counselling sessions, whilst some others do not. In the former, total duration of counselling turns out to be less time taking, as chances of misunderstanding remains minimal owing to the client's attitude and the parents' willingness to participate in an open discussion. However, counsellor has a significant role to play in preparing the parents to participate and developing an attitude in the client(s) to sit for joint session. In the former, chances of misunderstanding between the client and the parents remain high so long as the client does not agree to sit for open discussion jointly with the parents. In either case, however, initial plan of the counsellor to take individual sessions with the client(s) gets jeopardised, out of the demand of the situation to arrange for joint sessions.

In Indian culture mostly our parents have strong expectations to live in a joint family set-up with their sons and daughter-in-laws. Of late, many times, such expectation of the parents get jeopardised far several reasons, viz., daughter-in-law(s)'s unwillingness to stay jointly (where the son(s) is compelled to have a separate establishment), or on service ground sons have to be away from the parents, and so on. Such a situational demand which compels the son to remain separated from his parents acts as a failure on his part to provide necessary services to his parents; this he perceives as a personal shortcoming to keep up the expectation of his parents in particular and of his society at large. This causes severe guilt in the son—particularly when he is a strong believer of social norms and values. This in turn adversely affects his own family unit (constituting of his wife and children). Parents to considering our social norms, in some cases, become ashamed, as if, they have been rejected by their sons and daughter-in-law(s). Any individuals who fails to retain community standard (in some such way) experiences not only embarrassment of failure but severe guilt too, particularly seeing his parents ashamed.

Symptoms which our clients mostly develop—depression, OCD, hypochondriasis, and so on—are largely due to incongruities between their innate, registered social values and that of the acquired ones.

Some people engage in more maladaptive way of coping with negative emotions. They thus simply deny that they have any negative emotions and try to push those emotions out of conscious awareness. Such repressive coping may help individuals temporarily to prove that they are not in anyway 'bad', but becomes harmful both physically and psychologically in the long run. In our culture we very often comeacross clients with repressive coping. Individuals who are socially isolated face lot of conflicts in receiving social support if provided with. They are most likely to ruminate. Rumination leads to prolonged depression (Nolen-Hocksema and Larson, 1999). In our culture individuals with a tendency to ruminate, repeatedly talk about them having been involved in some activities which are unpardonable by the family in particular and his/her society, at large, but does not take any initiative to overcome ruminating habits. Initiative taking behaviour depends, by and large, upon one's social network. The client expects that social network would provide him support to ovecome problems. Social support becomes a proof to the client that he/she is pardoned (fuifilment of their needs to be acceptd and approved). Positive social suport may help people adjust better in stress by leading them to avoid ruminating about the stressor (Nolen-Hocksema, 1991). Thus, conflicted family relationship and social relationship, if any, becomes our main concern in counselling session.

People in India, particularly the older generation, is very strict in adhering to social norms and thus is highly sensitive to access to any deviation—whatever may be its modus operandus. In case of the latter, adjudication verdicts are mostly negative, i.e., to impose punishment on to the deviant. For example, in Indian culture, pre-marital and extra-marital sexual relationships, and consumption of alcoholic beverages are considered immoral. As such, even very occasional party drinking or history of infatuation during adolescence cause severe guilt in our clients much later in life. Such individuals manifest guilt-laden symptoms. These are some of the examples of conflicts which originate our of traditionalism versus modernism in our youth. Obviously, it possesses lot of dilemmas in our counsellor's too. Counselling, in such cases, requires focussing on such incongruities first, no matter what the nature of the client's presenting symptoms are. To probe into incongruities we are to depend on the client because the client at his stage requires to account for his/her current life situations including his/her interpersonal issues and available interpersonal resources, viz., family and social support network. This is typical of Indian set-up that even if a client realises his liabilities and assets through counselling (which is supposed to be enough to ameliorate his/her problem(s), as a last resort, the client usually expects support from his family to ensure his unconditional acceptance by them. Unconditional in the sense that guilt has been ingrained in the client through family upbringing process, the client expects that if unbiased acceptance by the family would mean that he/she is really forgiven for his/her past misdeeds. It appears as though self-realisation through counselling which the client has achieved so far remains incomplete till the client is provided with family/social support. Thus, group intervention strategy mostly comes in force as a model even if the counsellor intends to initiate individual intervention strategy. For clients like this, such strategy becomes inevitable to reach a state of relapse prevention.

Family support and support from the larger society becomes a key-source of reconciliation for our clients. It has been mentioned earlier in this write-up that lack of family support/social support has been found to be one of the major sources of behavioural problems in clients of this culture. Obviously, counselling of our clients requires a probe into this aspect of interpersonal interaction of our clients.

Model 4 : On Religious Issues

By and large, people in India believe in religion no matter what is the nature of the ethos they inherit. Visiting religious institutions to pay homages to the Almighty is, so to say, a daily life schedule here. A significant section of our population, when under emotional distress, visit religious centres to overcome distress. The religious places, as such, seem to have a power of healing (Raghuram, Venkateswaran, Ramkrishnan, and Weiss, 2012). Also, the leaders of such religious institutions/centres (designated differently in different religions) provide a strong support to the distressed by offering them some antidotes indigenous in nature (e.g., sacred oil, sacred water, roots of some plants and so on), which appear to have a pharmacological/medical impact onto the distressed. Incidentally, it may be mentioned here that in a survey in Tamil Nadu, South India, Campion and Bahugra (1996) found that about 40% of the psychiatric patients consulted a religious leader prior to their attending hospitals for consultation with a clinician/physician.

It is not within the purview of this book to go into a detailed description of the nature of different traditional healing methods recently being practiced in India, but enough research evidences are available to justify that the traditional healing methods have still now some medical implications in providing emotional support to the perturbed individuals—irrespective of the geographical area of this country the individuals hail from. Medical implications of such methods can be explained in a different perspective in context to Indian culture.

People of this country mostly believe in the medical model of treatment where the client is provided with a prescription by the respective physician. But problem arises particularly with regard to those clients who do require only counselling/psychotherapy, but no medication at all. In such instances too, the clients demand a prescription from the counsellor. For instance, a client said, "Dr., how is that you are planning for my treatment without providing me with a prescription?" The 'Prescription' term is used in two different meanings : (a) prescription means the patient is provided with a document which contains the personal information and related information about the illness; and (b) what all is discussd during counselling be summarised and handed over to the client in the form of a document (prescription). Some counsellors do provide their clients prescription like that of the latter kind. Sometimes, that client is convinced that such treatment is possible without any prescription, but the guardians of the client(s) insists upon the same. At this juncture, a contradiction appears. On the one hand, the client—even the guardians—claim that confidentiality be maintained strictly on personal information, on the other hand they insist upon providing them with a written document about the contents of the counselling sessions conducted. Providing such a document to the guardians sometimes puts the client in a more distressed condition (particularly when the client is not willing to disclose information in black and white to anyone), and sometimes personal information get disclosed through the relatives of the client and the client virtually gets a feedback of the same and starts accusing the counsellor. Such contradictions, however, provide the counsellor with some important cues about the client's environment, viz., possessiveness of the parents/guardians of the client, strong dependency need of the client onto a significant person in life, and so on. These issues are to be dealt with adequately during counselling proper. It must not mean that medical prescription as such has no importance in our life. Indeed it has, but only when it is essential. Unlike a medical practitioner, for a counsellor (who is a paramedical professional), it is not mandatory to provide the client with a prescription. This is to focus here as to how our clinicians/counsellors face additional problems at the very initial stage of counselling; convincing clients and their relatives takes time. Unless such preliminary issues are settled, counselling in real sense cannot be initiated.

When religious leaders provide the clients some antidotes, the antidotes become the object of dependency for our clients. The antidotes, i.e. the objects, shadow the leader. The procedures explained by the leader regarding the use of antidotes act as a prescription to our clients. When instructions during counselling, are provided with verbally, the clients become apprehensive that they might forget the steps to be followed. Likewise, in counselling sessions too, e.g., in cognitive therapy, when homework is assigned to them, the clients prefer a brief write-up from the counsellor, instead of verbal instructions. Such a write-up matches well with the client's existing cognitive scheme of obtaining a prescription from the consultant; otherwise homework, when assigned verbally to the client, is nothing but a prescription like the one provided by a physician about the dosages and duration of medicine. Psychologically, such a prescription-bound orientation of our clients during counselling reflects nothing but their lack of self-trust and lack of self-confidence in taking responsibilities onto themselves. Lack of self-trust raises doubts (insecurity) in the clients, at least initially, about the counsellor's commitment and, thus, a written document from the counsellor can ensure the clients in this regard. Providing with a written document means to them that they can retain their habit of being a follower rather than a leader; an issue which has to be dealt with carefully in the counselling sessions proper.

Because of such dependency, our counsellors most frequently get a query from their clients as to whether thy should continue the religious modes of intervention? The answer from the counsellor in this regard must be always in a non-commital fashion. The counsellor must not impose his/her belief system onto the clients. The counsellors' attitude must convey an indirect message to the clients that if different modes of intervention give satisfactory outcome, then the counselee should decide which mode to intervention give satisfactory outcome, then the counselee should decide which mode to continue. Of course, from clinician's viewpoint, the counsellor should advice the client(s) that follow-up of any method of intervention be done methodically to present relapse.

In corollary to what has just been depicted above, it may be stated that, of the two models of psychotherapy (Neki, 1973), namely, 'Guru-Chela' (teacher-pupil) relationship, and 'Sahaja' (togetherness) therapy, the former was found ideal for the Indian patients (the term 'patient' has been used by Neki), as was the observation of Neki. Togetherness implies a sense of responsibility and that is in terms of sharing with each other, whereas the teacher-pupil relationship implies that one (the pupil) can be made knowledgeable with assistance from the other (teacher), i.e. the pupil can depend upon the teacher. The reasons for the former models becoming popular (ideal) lies in our very upbringing style, which provides enough scope and indirect assurance to depend on the seniors/parents/superiors, especially for the matters related to decision-making . While establishing counselling/psychotherapeutic relationship with our clients/patients, such personality characteristics of our clients/patients are to be dealt with carefully; otherwise, it is likely to cause serious problems regarding the phenomenon of transference in counselling relationship. Our clients' dependency needs in general, and consequent expectations from the counsellor/therapist become the determining factors regarding clinicians' decision about the degree of lead to be taken by them during the sessions. Our clinicians are to be specially alert in handling such phenomena.

In continuation to what has been stated in the opening lines of this section that attitudinal differences prevail amongst our clients regarding psychosocial-religious issues which have significant impact in our therapeutic endeavour, it requires special mention that, of late, such attitudinal differences in matters related to religious beliefs are mostly noted in our society between the older generation and the younger, where the latter doesn't want to be a blind follower of what-all is advised by the seniors in this regard. For example, a boy of Class VIII reported to a counsellor that he doesn't find any justification in worshipping idols though he is constantly being nagged by his parents to do the same. The parents of the boy reported that the child is becoming very stubborn and displays a tendency to defy his parents, particularly for matters related to religion. The problem becomes more acute when the conflict becomes apparent between the parents of the child in similar issues. For example, a boy of Standard II (6 yrs) is found to be in a dilemma regarding formation of attitude towards religion. The child hails from a family where his father and paternal grandparents do not believe in religion (worshipping idols), whilst his mother and maternal grandparents are strong believers of the same. The source of dilemma in the child is six fold : (i) attitudinal differences between the parents of the child; (ii) attitudinal differences between the boy and his father; (iii) attitudinal differences between the boy and his mother; (iv) attitudinal differences between the paternal grandparents and maternal grandparents of the boy; (v) between the boy and his paternal grandparents, and that (vi) between the boy and his maternal grandparents.

As a consequence the boy has developed aggressive attitude towards his mother so much so that the boy in some occasions, particularly when mother request him to worship, has destroyed the idols in presence of his mother. To deal with the child's aggressive behaviour in the beginning, counselling with the parents is very essential. This is to help the parents develop that type of attitude which will be conducive for the child to exercise his own views and to re-think as to whether he finds any justification for his parents in insisting him upon to follow the directions given by them. Since the child will thus be provided with opportunities to exercise his own viewpoints independently, this will not create any retaliation in the child (immediate gain); on the other, it may even help him to realise in the long run as to how to avoid confrontation with his parents in this regard (long term gain). But our parents mostly fail to have patience. They are apprehensive that the child will be beyond their control if they do not intervene immediately. They start nagging him to follow their directions, which, in turn, is perceived by the child as interference in his independent decision-making. Having such a mental state (lack of freedom in decision-making) when the child attains adolescence, he/she shows behavioural problems like, excessive rigidity, tendency to defy the authority and the like. Parents' insecurity (whether the child be a model one) and related behaviour make the child confused at the formative stage of his/her development. Such conclusions later make the child victim of several behavioural problems.

A moot question arises concerning the extent of lead to be taken by the counsellor. The term 'lead' has different connotations (Robinson, 1950), description of which is beyond the scope of this chapter. However, the very essence of lead is degree of direction in communication. In this sense, silence is also a lead. Let us see now which type of communication is suitable for our clients in Indian cultural set-up. Silence (i.e., passive listening) does not encourage our clients. They mostly think that (i) they are not properly entertained by the counsellor; (ii) they further interpret the counsellor's lack of interest to take up the case; (iii) in some instances clients think a step further that perhaps his/her case is very complicated; (iv) the counsellor haven't come across similar cases before; (v) the counsellor fails to understand the genesis of the problem of this case, (vi) the methods to be implemented for counselling and so on, and (vii) thus, the counsellor is giving an indirect message that let the client leave him. This is so stated because, many a times the clients ask directly, "Dr., you haven't shown any reaction to my reporting; have you come across any such client before, do you think, Dr. that I can be cured?"

On the other hand, silence may mean that what all the clients reported, everything has been accepted by the counsellor without any censor. This should encourage the clients that they can convince the consultant through reporting. But usually, silence discourages our clients, as they feel insecured, thinking that the counsellor is not dependable. Such an arbitrary interpretation and or reflection of the clients' myopic view (mind's eye) about the whole course of intervention method to be applied by the respective counsellor. This, however, provides a sufficient cue to the counsellor that the client is impatient about his/her need fulfilment, i.e., need to depend.

In the client-centred approach, our clients mostly surrender to the counsellor stating that "Dr., I don't find any answer to your question about my complaints; you please tell me what it is about". Our clients hardly take a challenge to discover the hidden facts behind their ailments even when they are provided with cues to prove such factors. So, the very purpose of applying the client-centred approach is jeopardised. On the contrary, if a counsellor takes a direct lead, there too, many clients fail to understand implications of depth interpretation; many disagrees with the interpretations provided on some abstract concepts, and still many others, though they understand the implications of depth interpretation, show strong resistance to accept it. Nevertheless, some of the clients agree with depth interpretation and cooperate since beginning. The former problem would not arise if the counsellor can select a right technique for the right client. For the latter problems it is, of course, the duty of the counsellor to help the client to break resistance.

If the method of counselling is behaviourally oriented, many a times family members of the client and the client himself/herself fails to follow carefully the work schedule given with adequate motivation. Here, class is apparent mostly with a medical model of intervention. That is, clients mostly prefer to remain passive, like swallowing a medicine, as prescribed by the respective physician in a pharmacotherapy model, instead of taking a lead in undertaking responsibility which are required to implemen the behaviour therapy schedule assigned to them (for home situation) by the respective counsellor. Some of the clients, under such circumstances, comment like "Dr., can I not follow the schedule in your prescence only" (deserve continuous supervision), "instead of me and my family members taking the responsibility of implementing it in your absence". This shows that they demand a direct lead from the counsellor.

In cognitive restructuring model, it is mostly found that the clients show lack of motivation to finish homework assignments. "Dr., I won't be able to finish up the assigned work myself; you please help me to get rid of my problem quickly." Here too, they demand that the counsellor take a direct lead to solve their problems. At the same time an opposite picture of their mental status gets revealed when the counsellor desires to probe into some of the very core personal life events of the clients, viz., guilt, particularly sexual guilt, if any, complexes in personal life sphere of the clients, and so on. These clients, out of inhibition, resist communication on such related issues.

From the above statements, it is clear that our clients, by and large, are concerned about symptomatic relief; etiological understanding of the symptoms, does not pave way for treatment because of the clients non-cooperation, even though the counsellors intend to make the clients aware of the etiological bases of the reported symptoms. However, for a cross-section of the clients namely, the literate group, CBT, dynamic interpretation of symptoms, client-centred intervention strategies do work well, provided the counsellor can select a right technique for a given client. Otherwise, there may be a good beginning but incomplete end.

In fact, what, when, and whom etc. in selecting a mode of intervention can't be answered in a matter of fact way, or by applying a formula. Much of it depends upon the counsellors' clinical acumen, intuitive judgement, clinical expertise, and the nature of the problem reported by the clients. Every counsellor, through his/her expertise, may develop a technique of his/her own (with some modification of existing techniques) which may not strictly adhere to any classical intervention strategy. Culture-bound modifications of some of the existing classical techniques are also necessary. Every client is a new book. As such, no client seems to fit in well with all the inclusion-exclusion criteria reported in literature regarding applicability of a given intervention technique for a given client.

Contradictions in Counselling

Some clients do whilst some do not benefit from counselling. Medical treatment at times involves discomfort—and counselling, too, is no exception. Freud long ago reported that psychotherapy can cause negative effectives (Freud, 1923, 1961). However, percentage of clients who do not benefit from counselling is very low. In fact, if carefully assessed, it can be guessed prior to initiation of counselling as to who will profit from counselling/psychotherapy, which technique will suit best for a given client. Some negative factors act as contraindicators. Some such factors are—exacerbation of existing symptoms; appearance of new symptoms when amelioration of major symptoms take place at a satisfactory level, and so on. Of course, all negative symptoms are not contraindications. There is wide individual variation in attributing meanings to a given symptom. For instance, in some cases at the end part of the counselling programme, clients experienced depression out of guilt over some past deed. This is not really a contraindication—provided the client's conscience was inhibited till he/she joined counselling programme. Zetzel (1965) opined that depression might be a sign of progress in narcissistic personality. Likewise, ability to feel anxious in a client who was unable to experience anxiety, or who warded it off with denial may be considered a sign of progress (Zetzel, 1970), as decreased anxiety in a highly anxious client indicates progress. 'Negative therapeutic reaction' has been documented by Sandler, Dave and Holder (1992), where these authors reported that sometimes clients transiently feel worse despite therapeutic progress. This has been detailed earlier in this book.

Some of the reasons for (in addition to those in Chapter 11) negative effects in counselling include—inadequate diagnostic evaluation (wrong selection of test and incorrect assessment reports), inadequate training of the counsellor which might even lead to misapplication of counselling technique. Thus, to ignore altogether, in principle, the potentials for negative effects in and of themselves is erroneous because they may not at all contraindicate the therapeutic effect, they rather contraindicate (Cameron *et al*, 1998) certain therapeutic goals and techniques. For instance, explorative psychotherapy may induce certain stress in cases with PTSD (Krystal, 1988) as psychodynamic technique may lead to a psychotic transference (reality testing lost) in some patients with poorly defined boundaries (Kernberg *et al*, 1989).

Chapter 17

COUNSELLING : NEED FOR INTEGRATION

There are as many theoretical constructs and techniques of counselling that are already available to us. This creates dilemma in the counsellor as to which theoretical construct and its corresponding counselling technique will be appropriate for a given patient/client; to add to it all, many more new techniques are being proposed almost every year.

The dilemma takes an altogether different shape when we come across techniques which overlap in their theoretical constructs. For example, cognitive therapy (CT), and cognitive behaviour therapy (CBT) and rational emotive therapy (REBT). Ellis distinguishes REBT from CBT by putting emphasis on philosophy (Ellis, 1994). Ellis opined that CBT, though emphasises cognitive processes, does not have a specific philosophic emphasis, as REBT has. In REBT theory emotion is central. According to REBT theory, people make themselves emotional victims of their own irrational and unrealistic thinking patterns. So, goal of REBT is to help the clients make a philosophic change (Ellis, 1994) to control their present and future emotion and behaviour (pp. 241, 247). When Ellis talks about philosophic change, he means to say, perhaps, that the belief system of the client is formed through his philosophy in life and thus change in philosophy will bring a permanent change in the present belief system of the client.

Now the question arises, that if belief systems of the clients are the concrete operations of the formal abstract philosophy, then in CT/CBT also—when cognitive restructuring is the aim—then there too, cognitions cannot be restructured without touching upon the basic social philosophy of the client, which has helped him to form the present cognition (belief). In CT, when 'homework' is assigned to the client (to exercise his belief system with all pros and cons prior to taking a new decision) that is, perhaps, synonymous to Ellis' concept of 'philosophic change'. If a counsellor, in CT, for example, does not focus upon the roots that form cognitive constructs (i.e., belief system formed out of philosophy) of a given client, then that restructuring of cognition is incomplete and relapse is likely to occur. Such a decision on the part of the counsellor is again unexpected. The goal of counselling is to help the client change particular belief system (cognition) which has victimised the client emotionally, and thus to help him/her make decisions about his/her life style (cognitive-existential), and to act (behavioural) accordingly. Therefore, counselling in real sense requires integration of three basic philosophies—idealism, existentialism, and realism, no matter what is the technique the counsellor selects for a given client.

Attempts for integration poses a lot of problems to our clinicians. Problems which Indian clinicians usually face are really complicated and bidirectional in nature. Because, they are to help the clients ameliorate their problems which have been ingrained in them culturally, but by applying those techniques which have been largely adopted in different culture and that too from an altogether different perspective. As mentioned above, while cross-cultural differences reflect differences in basic philosophy of life, obviously our problems are unique in their own way—be it regarding marital disharmony, or educational or vocational or personal problems of the client. Though these problems can very well be designated under the general rubric of, say, marital disharmony or personal inadequacy, etc., the perspective in which counselling services are to be rendered here are quite different in nature. For example, counselling with gay/lesbian individuals, or with a divorcee, or with an individual having inadequacy, and so on. Some of the case vignettes are depicted below in order to help our students to have a clear understanding of this problem.

Case Vignettes

(I) Male, 24 yrs, unmarried graduate, employed, came for consultation mainly to clear off his doubts whether he can lead a satisfactory marital life since he has had no experience of sex as yet.

In Indian culture, to remain virgin till marriage (for both the male and female) is no wonder, though it may be perceived as unusual in some other cultures. Also, the clients' attitude towards sex at his premarital stage (i.e., to refrain from) is quite in the expected directions (as per the social norm).

The given client's problem is lack of confidence in himself. This is owing to apprehension of failure and subsequent social humiliation, though he is well motivated to maintain a heterosexual life style after marriage.

Suck lack of confidence is due to his incomplete and even incorrect knowledge about sex which he has gathered through some unauthentic magazines, and some such other sources. Also, sometimes friends have provided him knowledge in this regard which, once again, though incorrect, is strong enough to make him feel incompetent (apprehension of inadequacy). Conflict also arises when he has learnt that some males of his age are no longer virgin though as yet unmarried. In simple, his dilemma is—whether to go for marriage remaining virgin (social desirability), or to have a trial to have experience of sex before marriage to gain confidence (the latter induces severe guilt in him). In such a case, for the counsellor, the task is not that easy as it apparently sounds. The counsellor can never advise him to have a trial before marriage, nor can he assure him that in future he won't come across any experience of failure in this regard. If the former is advised the counsellor will be condemned by the parents of the client and also by the society, and, if the latter, the counsellor is not sure whether he/she would be balmed in any way in the future. It is advisable to refer the case for having thorough physical examination done and to complete other related investigations by the expert specialists in this arena. Counselling help would be to provide him assistance to regain confidence.

(II) Male (30 years), undergraduate, unmarried, now being insisted upon by his parents to get married (parents have selected match), came for consultation with the question whether he can lead a heterosexual life. He reported to having same sex interaction several times and also fantasises about having sex with male celebrities, although possesses occasional desire to change his life style (sexually). It is a matter of concern specific to this culture, as remaining unmarried till 30 years of one's life may be considered unusual, though usually persons in this culture do not agree to marry until they can become financially self-supported. One might think that since this guy had, had sex with males, so he is remaining unmarried. This is not necessarily true always; to remain unmarried, even otherwise, is not considered abnormal, if situation demands so. Likewise, arranged marriage even now is much in vogue (though love marriage is not that uncommon now).

Here, the client's orientation towards sex, though apparently seems heterosexual, poses strong desire for and orientation to the same sex interaction. He is not really motivated to change such orientation, though succumbs to parents' decision occasionally. He lacks determination in convincing parents (this causes lots of family unhappiness in Indian culture). Here the conflict is between social desirability (to comply with the parents) and lack of determination, lack of self-control, and competency (inadequacy).

Also some of the techniques for reframing sexual orientation depicted in the books of the origin of the West, are not applicable to Indian cultural set-up. This is not only in relation to gay or lesbianism, but in relation to sexual dysfunctions in married couples too. Obviously, some indigenous technique and/or integration of different techniques is required to suit the norms of this culture.

(III) Male, 27 yrs, marine engineer, in service, prospective groom, came for consultation, rather confirmation that he would be able to lead a happy conjugal life; the doubt which originates from conflicts related to his past sexual encounters. On enquiry it could be revealed that he had had sex with persons of the same sex (particularly in his place of occupation when he was placed abroad), but possesses strong inclination towards persons of the opposite sex. Homosexual relation is still a controversial issue in our culture, even though it may not be same in certain other societies.

Here the client's orientation towards sex gives a mixed picture; he better describes himself as an opportunist. That is, when person of the opposite sex are not available, he looks for persons of the same sex (bisexual?). Here conflict is between the choice of the object and socio-cultural norm. He is afraid, if any time his same sex relationship gets disclosed, he will have to face lot of social humiliation and embarrassment—both in his family as well as in his society.

(IV) Male, 30 yrs, undergraduate, unemployed, had had sex r 'ation with person of the opposite sex (always with the same person) though not yet married. He wants to avoid such relationship (due to social stigma) but fails. Being the only son of the family, parents have been insisting upon his marriage with a match of their choice.

Here the client has strong motivation to avoid this socially unacceptable sexual involvement; has strong desire to succeed in marital sexual life but is afraid of failure. In fact, further interview revealed that he has severe guilt conscience owing to have got involved in sex prior to marriage—as this is against Indian cultural norm. Associated with this is his fear of humiliation out of apprehension of getting such information disclosed in future, particularly to his wife. One way to assure him to overcome such guilt is to advise him to get married to that girl with whom he got involved in sex. Here too, as per Indian cultural norm, he is facing problems to make his parents convinced to arrange for marriage with this particular girl (though his parents aren't aware of his premarital involvement); on the other—and most strongest reason for his failing to convince his parents—is that he, too, doesn't like the girl really. If his society becomes aware of this, particularly the girl's side, then they will force him to get married to this particular girl only, because of his sexual relationship, no matter whether he dislikes the girl as his life partner. Disclosure of such facts to the parents will have severe hazardous consequences in the family, namely, even life threat. Here, the counsellor's dilemma is no less than that of the client, considering this cultural norm.

(V) Male, 29, undergraduate, unmarried, employed, no heterosexual exposure, reported that he requires assistance to decide upon his marriage. Enquiry revealed that the client had, during his early adolescence, sexual interaction with one of his hostel mates on persuasion by that person who was relatively senior to this client's age. The client did not like it, nor enjoyed it. This happened occasionally a few times. By nature the client is shy, unassertive, and sensitive about others' comments on him. Initially it caused problems in concentration and he had experienced deterioration in his academic performance for some time. He received counselling and could do well in subsequent examinations. He now wants to lead a normal marital life (heterosexual). Being the only son of the family, his parents also have been insisting upon his marriage. Here the client is in a constant conflict between avoidance of social stigma and conformity to social norm. On the one hand, he wants to marry (but apprehension of failure in conjugal life out of guilt for his past deeds, which also is causing a fear in him lest he be labelled as 'gay' by the society if he remains unmarried), on the other hand, he is equally perturbed, if he is unsuccessful to lead a marital life, he would be a failure to keep up his parents' expectation (social norm) through marriage. Mention needs be made here that remaining unmarried does not necessarily mean in this culture that the person is gay/lesbian. Such an apprehension in the given client is due to his guilt for getting involved in same sex relation. He can't accept it in a matter of fact way that it might happen for many in similar situations and at that age.

Let us examine now as to how differences are noted while applying counselling strategies across culture, though the basic theoretical construct of a given technique, and the complaints of the clients (at least apparently) remain same all over. Such difference in strategies are mainly due to the differences in the contents of the symptoms/complaints. REBT helps the client decide what he wants to do to solve a given problem, i.e., to see that the client can balance between logic and emotion while taking a particular decision.

From the above case illustrations it is clear that the genesis of the problems (and sex related phenomena) in these cases, thus, are largely a contribution of this culture. But all these clients do not possess the same level of motivation to deal with their problems. One has a strong motivation to avoid the stigma of being called 'gay', through marriage (vignette V), whilst another has a strong motivation to remain a 'gay' (vignette II); one is bisexual (vignette III) and wants to get married, and another is indecisive about marriage (vignette I), as he has had no experience of sex. In all the cases, some degree of guilt is present, but it is most severe in vignette IV (owing to pre-marital sex, though heterosexual in nature) and in vignette V (due to lack of knowledge that such casual relationships during adolescence does not necessarily make one homosexual in real sense). Such guilt-induced fear in all the cases is largely a product of this culture.

In sum, in the above case—sources of the problems are same whilst the nature and the intensity of the problems are widely diverse. Nature of the conflict is similar—i.e., failure to conform to social norms due to inadequacy (personality) but, at the same time, fear of othrs' comment (social stigma) and thus he/she succumbs to the situation against his/her will.

One might opine here that the problems which have so far been focussed by the author do not represent the entire panorama of the problems we come across in counselling in this culture, but rather a crossectional presentation, i.e., sex and sex related problems only. The global picture of problems which we come across in counselling set-up has already been mentioned in the previous chapters of this book, namely gender discrimination, parental upbringing processes, parental expectations, joint family atmosphere, etc., which are of cultural origin, and thus, these are not discussed here again. The purpose of highlighting the sex-related problems here is to focus upon, as an e.g., the difficulties of application of Western counselling strategies in our counselling set-up. This is because sex and sex related knowledge, ideas, imaginations, guilt etc. are mostly found to be present as genesis of majority of the problems reported, particularly by our adolescents and young adults. Otherwise, the problem of inadequacy, marital discord or fear of failure in exam, for example, is not unique in a particular culture.

The variation in symptom manifestation is due to the meaning of the symptom/complaints as determined by a given culture. Accordingly, counselling strategies need to be modified to best suit this culture. Foulks long ago (1980) pointed out that culture provides guidelines and rules not only for recognising and diagnosing emotional problems/illnesses, but also for its management/treatment. Criticisms have been directed against professional clinicians who fail to explore the role of culture in the diagnosis of mental illness (Fernando, 1991; Pinderhughes, 1989). Similar criticisms might be labelled at those psychotherapists/clinical counsellors who fail to apply cultural factors in selecting and implementing their therapeutic/counselling strategies (Gibbs, 1985). Not only normalcy and deviancy, but degree of recovery from illness and/or symptom amelioration too need be evaluated through the cultural lens of the society. As already mentioned earlier in this book that culture is not a monolith; and individual client/patient at times may be influenced by more than one culture. Thus, psychosocial factors, individual history, circumstances and the institutional (does not mean a hospital-like institution but refers to a culture) systems in which the therapist/counsellor and the patient/client work is of crucial (Gibbs, 1985) importance.

Secondly, independent decision-making is encouraged in the West. Therefore, if one wants to enjoy his life as gay, he doesn't feel ashamed, nor feels pressurised from the family to change his life style and to get married etc. In contrast, in the Indian society, a gay or lesbian feels segregated from the mass and is somehow ashamed and feels awkward if identified even now. However, compared to the past, more number of such individuals are responding/receiving counselling services to deal with social and personal desires. As decision-making, particularly regarding education and marriage, becomes predominantly a collective phenomenon in this culture, individuals with sexual problem, and for the matters related to their marriage, face lots of problem in deciding upon their life style. Similar problems occur, in some cases, with regard to deciding upon the clients' choice of academic specialisation. Obviously such hesitation on the part of the client on the one hand, and persuasion on the part of his family members on the other cause hindrance to get quick counselling/therapeutic outcome. If one follows case illustrations and the mode of therapeutic intervention of Ellis (1971), e.g., it is evident that Ellis is non-judgmental about the life-style issues of the clients. He argued and urged that the client should make a decision based on personal preference, rather than "absolute must", and to learn to live with that decision comfortably. In client-centred approach, technically speaking the counselling must be non-judgemental. Likewise, personal preference in decision-making is likely to produce relatively less stress in the decision-maker. But in Indian set-up—remaining non-judgemental, at times, becomes difficult for the reasons mentioned before. Regarding personal choice in decision-making in this culture, it is found that the clients—even though understand well their personal preferences (emotion)—remain indecisive about their social acceptance (can't reason out as per social norm). Thus, in Indian set-up, the basic dependent nature of the client and the subsequent indecisiveness make them vulnerable to depend totally on the counsellor.

To prevent relapse, integration between emotion and thinking is very essential. The clients start feeling that they are bad, and not liked by the society. "I'm a gay, I'm bad". "I'm incompetent to satisfy my parents' expectation through marriage with a match of their choice, so I'm not desired at all now by my parents", and so on. If the counsellor has to attack the client's belief system or deal with the unfoundedness of those beliefs, the counsellor has to face lots of resistance—both from the client as well as from his family members. Question may arise that why not start with individual counselling only in such cases? Again, the problem the counsellor has to face here is, what is already mentioned above, that the clients' decision in such cases is largely a collective act. In some cases, the client seeks help from the counsellor that if the counsellor can convince him/her parents to comply with the client's preference in maintaining his/her life style, which may not be in congruence with that of the parents' decision. In Indian set up, the counsellor is again in a dilemma at this stage of counselling. The counsellor's prime focus is to help the client develop self-confidence so as to get rid of all irrational fears; on the other, if such a decision is not in congruence with that of the client's family members', that can even lead to very dangerous consequences for the family. The latter also, in turn, causes severe distress in the client. This is, thus, altogether a different situation in this culture compared to that of the West. Therefore we need to have our own indigenous methods of counselling strategies. But to make the client decisive about his life style in the above-cited cases, client-centred orientation, takes lots of time and the clients do not feel encouraged to continue counselling as they want immediate outcome. However, exceptions are also evident. Gay individuals in our society unfortunately adopt oppressive ideas from the society. This belief system, in turn, results in a negative self-image, and personality inadequacy. Some such client want to prove to the society that they are heterosexual in life style though they really are not. Such defence causes hindrance in the initial few sessions of counselling progress. However, the counsellor has to be sure first whether the client is using any such defense and to formulate counselling strategy accordingly. Therefore, the interview style of Ellis (1971) may be suitable for a given culture (Ivy *et al*, 1997), but not universally for all different cultures. Modification of a technique and synthesis of some are necessary to overcome such confrontations and cognitive discrepancies in our clients which have been engraved in them through the culture they belong to.

In sum, this chapter addresses the role of culture with respect to some of the elements of counselling practice and thereupon need for integration of the techniques to adhere to our social norms and customs.

Chapter 18

GOALS OF COUNSELLING

Counselling to be effective has to be specific for each client as each client has unique problems and expectations. Accordingly, the goals of counselling would also be different in nature, namely, immediate versus long-term, process versus specific. Whatever it may be, goals of counselling must be clear to the client since it provides a direction and purpose. Goals can establish a congruency between the client's expectation and what and how much of it he can be provided with practically by the counsellor.

The process goals, as the name implies, are concerned with effectiveness of the techniques/procedures that can facilitate counselling outcome. Process goals comprise of essential counselling conditions, viz., empathic understanding and warmth required for interpersonal exploration. Specific goals, on the other hand, are problem-centred. It is concerned with the client's problems, client's expectations, client's cognitive assets and liabilities, and other environmental resources available to help the client with reference to the specific issues under consideration.

Immediate goals refer to the problem(s) which require, (the client needs) immediate resolution. In this sense, it is concerned with the here-and-now phenomenon of the problems. Every here-now-now problem has/is supposed to have a root which requires time to reveal and restructure. From this point of view, immediate goal may be considered as a step to long-term-goal. Complete self-understanding through self-exploration, though aimed at, may not be possible in immediate goal seeking procedure, as because the client has to be counselled on the issue under reference immediately. At best, the client may be helped and made to understand his strengths and weaknesses in such sessions; it may be more of an information providing session, but configuration of such information would not be possible unless the client has an integrative understanding of himself, his personal resources, vis-à-vis his environmental resources and constrains. Such integration and resolution of the self require long time.

Long-term goals, thus, aim at helping the counselee to attend self-actualisation, self-realisations, and self-enhancement. Goals of counselling may appear to differ depending upon the nature of the goals (immediate or long term, specific or process) as well as depending upon the orientation of the counsellor (behaviourally oriented—

stress the need for behaviour modification; Growth oriented—stress the need for development of inner potentialities; Existentially oriented—stress the need for self-enhancement; Dynamically oriented—stress the need for personality restructuring etc.). However, each of these, again, have some common goals. These are—(i) to help the client learn to make decisions independently through best utilisation of available intrapersonal and interpersonal sources; (ii) to improve personal effectiveness (through impulse control and conflict resolution); (iii) to find solution to problems independently (through developing insight), and, thus (iv) to achieve positive mental health (through coping with tension, frustration; and promotion of psychological well-being (developing respect for oneself as well as for the self of others), and thus to become a fully functioning individual. In this sense, all the above-mentioned goals may be supplementary to each other.

Mention needs be made that, like any intervention strategy, counselling also is not free from limitations. It may not be universally applicable to all irrespective of the nature of the problem reported. It is not a panacea.

In short : The goal of counselling is to help the client gain :

(i) Understanding one's own limitations (U)

(ii) Discovering one's own assets/potentiality (D)

(iii) Accepting responsibilities (A)

(iv) Independent decision-making and action (I)

(v) Prepared to face the consequences of action (P)

(vi) Understanding the consequences (meaning) of the action (U)

(vii) Restructuring cognitive frame of reference (R).

Thus, the counsellor helps the client to discover the silver lines from gloomy past of his life; he/she reaches UDAIPUR.

Chapter 19

PREVENTION OF STRESS

Until now, focus had been on intervention, however, prevention of any illness is of high priority than its treatment, so also for stress-related disorders. Prevention may be primary, secondary, and tertiary. Primary prevention aims to develop techniques to stave off stress disorders from individuals who are currently healthy. Secondary prevention targets high risk individuals to forestall illness and also to lessen the chances of replace in remitted cases. Tertiary prevention aims to promote health—both physical and psychological—and thus it focuses upon development of more sensitive and responsive management, e.g., implementation of occupational health schemes and family support provisions and similar other plans, follow-up programmes for maintenance of such provisions and enhancement of services through research (to promote health).

Leka & Griffiths (2005) have provided a succinct view of all three types of prevention in context to work stress. According to them, primary prevention includes ergonomics (use of updated sophisticated equipments and better facilities), work and environmental design (improved physical working conditions, and work scheduling), and high organisational and management development (to improve managers' attitude to deal with workers in understanding their problems promptly). Secondary prevention, they suggested, is through worker education and training, and tertiary prevention comprises of development of overall management system though implementation of better occupational health provisions to reduce recurrence of stress related problems. Of these three modes, they have emphasised more on the tertiary mode of prevention. A comprehensive programme of work-stress prevention would now be described.

A. PRIMARY

(i) Modified methods be employed for selection and recruitment

One of the important factors of job stress is 'role ambiguity' and/or 'role conflict' in the workers. To avoid this, recruitment methods must employ tools for accurate assessment of cognitive potentialities on the one hand, and personality characteristics of the workers on the other. The former includes assessments of creative potential related to the concerned work, and the latter includes assessment of leadership qualities, attitudes towards and involvement with the job and the organisation, responsibility taking behaviour, nature of interpersonal interaction with others etc. so that job placement and worker potentialities match well to enable the workers' adequate role execution.

Most updated modified tools, especially psychological tools, be employed for assessment of vulnerability if any, existing in the employee (to be selected) towards 'psychological contract' violation. Such violation may occur, either due to the employee's over-sensitivity towards organisation's promises, or the organisation's failure to uphold their commitments. Thus, care be taken that the 'psychological contract' is retained well to avoid stress. Both these are contraindication for stress free work environment.

(ii) Organisational environment be healthy and stimulating

Environment here refers to both physical environment, viz., work-place environment—its light, air, comfortable sitting arrangement and so on, and psychological environment, i.e., congenial employer-employee relationships. Adequate supervision needs be available when required. This must not be a mere official 'as-if' relationship, rather a relationship which reflects sharing and supportive attitude towards each other. Such an attitude helps developing 'we' feeling between them. Misbehaviour to the extent of bullying, harassing—from either side—must not be encouraged. The latter generates feeling of isolation in the individual, which is detrimental to overall production output of the organisation.

(iii) Organisations be aware of and concerned with the psychological sources of resentment in the employees

In addition to employer-employee and employee-employee relationships, and nature of pay package, job characteristics are also to be considered important in causing resentment. For example, under-stimulating, repetitive, non-creative works induce monotony in the workers. Possible ways and means to help employee overcome such monotony be thought of by the employer, e.g., rotation system in job assignment amongst the workers of the same status. Rotation and/or shifting duty system is required, but attention should be given to distribution of working hours amongst the workers in unbiased way. If possible, to allow the workers to avoid work during the period of unsocial hours, namely, late night shifts for consecutive weeks. Attention must also be given to equal distribution of work-load amongst the workers of a given status. Such scheduling can be perceived by the employees as flexible and fair—this reduces stress in them.

(iv) Assessment

To combat risk of stress, at source, the organisation should arrange for the following assessments : (1) to assess the risk of stress related to the work, and (2) to assess the risk of stress sourcing from the personality of the employee.

Normally these are done through standardised questionnaires. But questionnaire measures have certain definite limitations, viz., faking possibilities, inhibitions, hesitations on the part of the employee to reveal the actual feeling and, at times, inability of the employee to quantify his feelings through questionnaire measures. Indirect measures, viz., instruments may be used, e.g., lie-detector and the like to identify imbalance, if any, between the nature of work, pressure of work, and personal resources of the workers.

Organisational strategies for stress management should address risk assessment (exploration), planning, prevention, and executing the same. Such assessment is essential for designing rehabilitation programmes. Reevaluation is equally important to avoid future hazards.

(v) Organisations can arrange for team work for evaluation and management of stress

Team spirit helps better to comprehend a problem comprehensively. Organisations may differ in constituting a team, i.e.,., how to select the personnel who would comprise of a team? Perhaps it would be better if organisations comprehend a group which is comprised of representatives from the organisations' administrative level, finance representatives, HR personnel, medical unit specialists (specialist consultant physicians), and specialist consultant counsellors, psychologists), work supervisors, and employees' leaders, if any, and so on. Exchange of views amongst the representatives in a team provides clues for better understanding of the problems of both the employers and employees which, in turn, readuces resentment towards the authority.

B. SECONDARY

(i) Regular health check-up facilities be readily available at the work centre itself

Regular health check-up, both physical and psychological (particularly tension, worries, insecurities, personality problems which disturb work output), if can be made mandatory for the workers by a given organisation, would help not only for early identification of their problems but also would prevent them from future damage. At the time of recruitment, the workers must be informed about the availability of consultancy services by specialists, at the organisation itself, so that they can consult the respective specialists as per their need. It is advisable that strict confidentiality be maintained regarding those workers who consult psychiatrists/clinical psychologists/counsellor psychologists for their personal problems.

My personal experience in working as a consultant clinical psychologist-counsellor in corporate organisations show that employees are reluctant to come for psychiatric consultation which may be due to some social inhibition, viz., stigma. Accordingly, programmes for educating employees to overcome their resistance in this regard should be arranged for. Such consultations must always be arranged in one-to-one sessions only, and not in a group. Organisation also should develop an attitude not to be curious to know about personal information of the employees that get revealed to the consultants. If unusual event of an overt manifestation of a behavioural problem occurs, it could be dealt with as an exception by conjunct effort of the organisation and the consultant concerned. There, too, confidentiality should be maintained as far as practicable for future safe-guard of the client. 'Employee assistance programme' as Leka & Griffiths (2005) suggested, needs be implemented. Regular monitoring of health related problems and work-related issues would enhance level of satisfaction of the workers.

(ii) People management training programme for the supervisors and psychosocial stress-related management programmes for HR personnel

This is recommended so that the employees can get a prima facie support which helps them to combat stress—at least at the initial stage through the organisation's personnel (Leka & Griffiths, 2005). Training programmes are required to enlighten the participants for early detection/identification of behavioural problems, which, if not cared for immediately, might develop into major problems for the employees in future, as aftermath of prolonged stress. Supervisors and other committee members of the same status be provided with knowledge of 'first aid' assistance, on the one hand, and, on the other, knowledge about referral sources for subsequent care by specialists, if required. This would enhance employees' satisfaction. Also, members of the committee should be ready to enquire from the employees' family members whether any signal regarding behavioural problems of employee they have detected. For example, excessive use of alcohol, drug abuse or gambling and so on. Such dysfunctional coping behaviour should be addressed through comprehensive stress management programme (CSMP) (Hecker & Thorpe, 2005). Substance abuse can cause severe liver damage, hypertension, heart disease, brain dysfunctions—and even cancer. CSMP, depending upon the severity of the case, decides about referral of the case to specialist consultant for de-toxification programme, and/or for counselling. For other cases who require physical methods of treatment, namely, pharmacotherapeutical, anaerobic and aerobic exercises, be referred to the respective specialists. Physical exercises and meditation helps to reduce anxiety, high blood pressure, etc. Counselling helps to enhance self-esteem. Usually, resistant clients are found to be irregular in receiving counselling assistance; in such cases family assistance is required. Supervisors and committee members should have appropriate information and training on worker's health issues and on availability of health promoting support (Leka & Griffiths, 2005).

(iii) Organisations be concerned with enhancement of group morale of the workers

Both direct and indirect involvement with the organisation enhance group morale of the workers. Group morale provides a psychological boost-up to the workers. Direct involvement provides opportunities for (a) free interaction with the supervisors, and (b) participation in decision-making process. Respective supervisors should talk to their staff and allow them for free expressions of their problems and feelings about the organisation. The workers must be ensured that they have been given 'patient-hearing' by the organisation. Supervisors must not be egoistic with a sense of omnipotent and omniscience, thinking that their impressions about employees' feelings and thoughts are the last words. At times they also fail to understand employees' problems in true sense. From this develops a feeling of 'psychological contract violation' in the employees (Rousseau, 2004), which reduces group morale. Likewise, participation in decision making process enhances responsibility sharing attitude in the workers. This has been detailed in this chapter before.

(iv) To arrange awareness programmes for management personnel

Such programmes are necessary for the managers, group leaders, project leaders, supervisors and such others, so that they can easily detect signs of psychological problems, if any, which has developed in the employees due to work and work-place stress. This can function in a two-tier system : (a) the management personnel can refer the associates (employees) to the HR without any delay; and (b) the HR can provide first-aid services, thereafter, if necessary, can refer the associate to a specialist consultant. Thus group leaders, project leaders, supervisors and the like should be knowledgeable to detect and refer the clients to the HR for further necessary action (Nowack & Wimer, 2011). Health monitoring services provide security and psychological satisfaction to the workers (Leka & Griffiths, 2005).

(v) Work-family balance

Mostly employees fail to balance between work-pressure and family demands and needs. Usually long hours at work create family conflict. Expanded work week and sudden unconsented change in work schedule increases conflict with the family members. Internal work culture, viz., perceived inequalities in providing incentives and promotions to the workers, creates a revolting attitude in the latter towards the organisation. But the employees cannot expresses their resentment directly to the organisation. As a result, their suppressed resentment and aggression get displaced onto the innocent family members in the form of irritability, loss of temper, lack of interest in interaction with family members, particularly children, and also fatigue as a result of inadequate sleep and depression. The work-family balance struggle makes the employee physically and mentally exhausted. This has serious consequences with respect to accidents and poor performance in workers and distressed interpersonal relationship at the home front. The whole process tends-to-go in a cycle, placing the employee in a frying pan-to-fire situation.

Despite the existence of work-family balance policies in many organisations, there are some who discourage maintenance of such programmes in the work situations —at least indirectly. This occurs out of perceived inequalities in relation to work-schedule and work-promotion decided by the management. Nowack & Wimer (2011), in this context, reported that "rewards and promotions to those who put in the requisite amount of 'face time', staying at the office long enough to show they are good dedicated corporate citizens".

C. TERTIARY

(i) External sources for management of stress

In addition to reducing psychological distress, viz., anxiety, depression, etc., social support has been associated with lower incidence of onset of illness, and faster recovery from the illness. Social support has beneficial effects on the psyche and consequently on the physiological system of the individual, namely, on endocrine and immune systems and can reduce cardiovascular reactivity in stress (Uchino & Garvey, 1997).

Social support

Social support acts as an important source of stress moderator. It refers to all those resources that one can obtain through interaction with others. Interactions include, on the one hand (a) family members and relatives, viz., a network of communications and mutual obligations to each other, and, on the other (b) interaction with the larger society as well, viz., from the friends, clubs, religious institutions and so on (Siegel, 1993).

At the work place one may enjoy the emotional support of colleagues to reduce stress. Likewise, at the home front, he can share his burden of responsibilities, by discussing these with others. Maddi & Kobasa (1984) long ago reported that executives facing high level of stress appear to benefit from family support when they can prepare themselves to share their feelings and family members also understand and interact with them with a sharing attitude. Family support provides a feeling to them that they are part of a cohesive family in which they can freely express their emotions. Social-support helps reducing manifestations of symptoms—both physical and psychological.

There exists a great deal of individual differences in seeking social support as stress buffer. Typical introverts usually fail to avail of such resources. Sometimes such individuals though require sharing personal and emotional problems with others, they become status conscious (particularly managers and high officials) and they refrain from such interaction with colleagues and/or boss. Due to suppression of emotional problems they later suffer from several stress related disorders. The problem turns out to be more acute when they dislike sharing their personal problems with their family members too. They need to be trained to develop positive attitude towards seeking social-support to ameliorate stress. Usually individuals with lower social anxiety and better self-disclosure skills can utilise more social support to combat with stress.

Social support may be of several forms : appraisal support, tangible assistance, information and emotional support (Taylor, 1999) :

Appraisal Support : As the term implies, this technique of social support helps an individual to evaluate both the magnitude of the stressor as well as availability of coping resources. Suggestions from others and exchange of views with others about the actions to be taken may be more profitable than taking decision one self.

Tangible Assistance : This is to provide material support. For example, financial asistance and the like. .

Informational Support : This involves provision for both receiving a priori information from or providing information to the individual under stress well before he decides upon any action. For instance, seniors out of their work experience provide information to the juniors. For example, an young (24) associate of a corporate organisation was facing severe stress in dealing with his office boss, where the latter had used abusive language to the associate even in front of others at the office. When he came for counselling he was advised to enquire whether his seniors have been victimised like him, and to get information from them as to why that boss utters unparliamentary words and how they could minimise the situation. Such information seeking helped the concerned guy to overcome stress—at least temporarily. Then the associate was taken for individual counselling sessions.

Emotional Support : Prolonged and/or severe stress at times leads to emotional breakdown. Several symptoms may develop, viz., anxiety, depression, phobia and so on. Only close friends, relatives and family members can share the distress by providing support, security and assurance to the victims. Caregiver's active participation, in this sense, should be regarded as one of the best resources to rescue the individual under distress. The distressed individual develops a 'we' feeling and can overcome his loneliness and isolation.

Thus it is evident from the above that comprehensive programme for prevention of stress—be it primary, secondary, or tertiary—takes place through (1) individual counselling (psychotherapy), (2) in the form of group demonstration at work place (e.g., workshops), and (3) comprehensive employee assistance programmes. Each of these modes of prevention has been delineated separately in this book.

For individuals who require to attend special clinics for psychological assistance, the above-mentioned types of prevention are applicable—though their nature varies. In case of primary prevention, to save individuals from psychological distress, attempts are required to be taken for early detection of the nature and intensity of the problem through various assessments. Also, equally important is that to approach the respective clinician or hospital outdoor facilities at the earliest so as to prevent deterioration.

Secondary prevention includes regularity in following prescribed treatment/ therapeutic programme, be it psychiatric, pharmacotherapy, counselling/psychotherapy, or a combination of both, as the case may be, so as to avoid sporadic use of treatment. If otherwise, the progress of disease is likely to be enhanced rapidly, leading to poor prognosis. Follow-up is essential for each and every case to prevent relapse. These require active family support, especially for the reluctant patients.

Tertiary prevention aims at awareness programmes—both at the individual and family level—regarding genesis and manifestation of psychopathology. Though several NGOs, other private organisations, and mass media are providing support in this regard, a policy awareness programme should be organised, and directed at the government level. The Mental Health Act may have to be modified, particularly to provide adequate recognition to the psychologists whose services are mandatory for dealing with such type of problems.

Particular programmes need be taken up with the help of psychiatric social workers for home visit of clients/patients with psychological problems, so that available service facilities in this regard— both outdoor and indoor—could be readily available to the sufferers.

Counselling and psychotherapy, as methods of treatment/problem amelioration is applicable for individuals attending clinicies. However, thoice of treatment method would largely depend upon the psychopathology of the case.

Counselling methods, and its relation to psychotherapy, have been delineated in this treatise to the extent that they are applicable to both corporate sectors and clinics. However, there, are certain techniques which are specific to clinics—they have been mentioned briefly, as detailing of those appears beyond the scope of this book.

REFERENCES

Ackerman, N. (1970). Family interviewing : The study process. In N. Ackerman, Lieby, M. & Peurce, J. (Eds.), *Family Theory in Transition.* Boston : Little Brown.

Adler, N. & Mathews, K.A. (1994). Health and Psychology : Why do some people get sick and some stay well? *Annual Review of Psychology, 45,* 229-259.

Ahiaq, E. (1991). Enhanced therapeutic skills : Family & ethnic dynamics. Part I. *Paper presented at the North Atlantic Association for Counsellor Education & Supervision.* Albany : NY.

Alberti, R.E. & Emmons, M.L. (1995). *Your perfect right : A guide to assertive living.* Sun Luis Obispo, CA : Impact.

Alexander (1979). Rural psychotherapeutic process. In Kapur, M., Murthy, V.N., Sattyavathi, K. & Kapur, R.L. (Eds.). *Psychotherapeutic Process, NIMHANS :* Bangalore.

American Psychiatric Association (1980). *Diagnostic & Statistical Manual of Mental Disorders (3rd Edn.), Washington,* D.C.

American Psychological Association (1956). The Objectives of Counselling. *American Psychologists, 11,* 282-285.

Andrew, G., Dias-Saxena, F. & Patel, V. (2000). The development of a counselling treatment for common mental disorders in general health care settings. *Indian Journal of Clinical Psychology, 21(1),* 72-79.

Ang. S., van Dyne, L. and Beghey, T.M. (2005). The employment relationships of foreign workers versus local employees : a field study of organizational justice, job satisfaction, performance and OCB. *Journal or Organizational Behaviour, 24,* 561-583.

Applèy, M.H. & Turnbull, R. (Eds.) (1986). *Dynamic of Stress : Physiological, Psychological, and Social Perspectives,* New York Plenum.

Argyris, C. (1960). *Understanding organizational behaviour,* Dorsey Press, Homewood, IL.

Balodhi, J.P. & Mishra, H. (1983). Meditation as behaviour therapists view. *Behaviour Therapists, 6*, 196-197.

Bandura, A. (1989). Human agency in social cognitive theory. *American Psychologists, 44*, 1175-1185.

Banerjee, P. & Chattopadhyay, P.K. (2004). Depression : Role of control and defence variables. *Social Science International, 20(1)*, 33-42.

Barlow, D.H. & Durland, V.M. (2005). *Abnormal psychology : An integrative approach.* 4th ed., Pacific Grove, CA : Brooks, Cole Thompson Learning.

Basu, J. & Banerjee, M. (1998). Adaptation of the English version of the Ego Function Assessment Scale (modified). By Bellack for Indian Adults. *Indian Journal of Clinical Psychology, 25(1)*, 57-65.

Basu, J., Banerjee, M. & Mukhopadhyay, P. (1996). Applicability of the Ego Functions Assessment Scale on College Population. *Indian Journal of Clinical Psychology, 23*, 40-46.

Basu, S. (1994). *Integral education : Psychological Perspectives.* Bharat Printing, Kolkata.

Beck, A.T. (1997). Cognitive Therapy : Reflections. In J.K. Zeig (Ed.), *The Evolution of Psychotherapy.* The 3rd Conference, New York : Brunner/Mazel.

Beck, A.T. & Weishaar, M. (1995). Cognitive Therapy. In R.J. Corsini & D. Wedding (Eds.), *Current Psychotherapies, Zasca* : F.F. Peacock Publishers.

Begart, G. (1991). Meditation from transpersonal perspective. *American Journal of Psychotherapy, 45(3)*, 383-412.

Bhaduri, S. & Chattopadhyay, P.K. (1994). Psychalgia : A Study on the impact of stress. *Social Science International, 4*, 11-16.

Bhandari, A., Upamanyu, V.V. & Goyal, G. (2002). Correlates of depressive symptomatology at different levels of stressful life events. *Indian Journal of Clinical Psychology, 29(1)*, 19-23.

Bhatnagar, J. (2007). Talent management strategy of employee management in Indian IT employees : Key to relation. *Employee Relations, 29(6)*, 640-663.

Bhattacharya, J.P. (1986). *Psychalgia : Ethno-psychiatric knowledge in Bengal.* Foreign & Comparative Studies/South Asian Services. New York : Syracuse University.

Bhola, P. & Kapur, M. (2000). Prevalence of emotional disturbance in Indian adolescent girls. *Indian Journal of Clinical Psychology, 27(20)*, 217-222.

Biswas, A., Biswas, D. & Chattopadhyay, P. K. (1995). Cognitive behaviour therapy in Generalized Anxiety Disorder. *Indian Journal of Clinical Psychology, 22(2)*, 1-10.

Biswas, A. & Chattopadhyay, P.K. (2002). Cognitive therapy in GAD : Psychological and physiological outcome. *Indian Journal of Clinical Psychology, 27(2)*, 192-199.

Bose, R. (1997). Psychiatric and popular conception of possession among the Bangladeshis in London. *International Journal of Social Psychiatry, 43*, 11-15.

Bosma, H., Marmot, M.G., Hemmingway, H. *et al* (1997). Low job control and risk of coronary heart disease in Whitehall II (Prospective Cohort) Study. *British Medical Journal, 314*, 285.

Bowlby, J. (1988). *A secure base.* New York : Basic Books.

Brammer, L.M. & Shostrom, E.L. (1968). *Therapeutic Psychology : Fundamentals of actualization counselling & psychotherapy.* Englewood Cliffs, N. J. Prentice-Hall.

Brayfield, A.H. (1961). Vocational guidance today. In P.G. Williamson (Ed.), *Vocational counselling : A reappraisal in honour of Donald G. Patterson.* Minnesota Studies in Student Personnel Work. Vol. II, Minneapolis, Minnesota University Press, pp. 22-56.

Brayfield, A.H. (1963). *Counselling Psychology : An Annual Review.* Palo Alto, Annual Review, 14.

Bromberger, J.T. & Matthews, K.A. (1996). A longitudinal study of the effects of pessimism, trait anxiety, and life stress on depressive symptoms in middle-aged women. *Psychology & Aging, 11*, 217-223.

Buber, M. (1970). *I and thou.* New York : Scribner's.

Cameron, P., Ennis, J. & Deadman, J. (1998) (Eds.). *Standards and guidelines for the psychotherapies*, University of Toronto Press, Toronto.

Campaion, J., & Bhugra, R. (1996). Experiences of religious healing in psychiatric patients in South India. *Psychiatric Epidemiology, 32*, 215-221.

Cannon, W.B. (1932). *The Wisdom of the Body*, New York : Norton.

Carkhuff, R. (1969). *Helping and human relations* (Vols. 182), Troy, M.O. Holt, Rinehart & Winston.

Carstaris, G.M. (1965). Cultural element in response to treatment. In de Renek, & Porter, P. (Eds.), *Ciba foundation symposium on Transcultural Psychiatry*, J.A. Churchill Ltd., London.

Chakraborty, S., Saha, S., Mukhopadhyay, P., Chattopadhyay, P.K. & Biswas, D. (2001). Swimming and anxiety amelioration in children. A study using self report and physiological indices. *Bangladesh Journal of Sports Science, 1(1)*, 44-53.

Chatterjee, R. & Chattopadhyay, P.K. (2004). Asthma : Role of competition stress. *Social Science International, 20(1)*, 62-68.

Chattopadhyay, P.K. (1981a). Bilateral skill resistance response in anxiety. *Indian Journal of Clinical Psychology, 8(1)*, 29-34.

Chattopadhyay, P.K. (1981b). Application of a psychological technique in the treatment of Examination Phobia. *Society & Medicine, 10(2)*, 4-5.

Chattopadhyay, P.K. (1983). Bilateral EEG evoked response in anxiety. *Indian Journal of Clinical Psychology, 10(1)*, 151-157.

Chattopadhyay, P.K. (1998). Assessment of cognitive potentialities : A neuropsychological approach. In A. Sen & A. Sen (Eds.), *Challenges of contemporary changes : A psychological perspective on future human society.* New Age International Publication, New Delhi, pp. 73-92.

Chattopadhyay, P.K. (2009). Clinical Psychology in India. In Mishra, G. (Ed.), *Psychology in India : Revisited.* Fifth ICSSR Survey of Psychology (1993-2003). Chapter 20, Pearson Education, New Delhi.

Chattopadhyay, P.K., Bhaduri, S., Basu, A.K. & Basu, T.K. (1990). Psychalgia : A study of some personality factors. *Indian Journal of Clinical Psychology, 17(2),* 74-78.

Chattopadhyay, P.K. & Biswas, P.K. (1981). A psychological technique in the treatment of Writers' Cramp. *Society & Medicine, 10(2),* 2-3.

Chattopadhyay, P.K. & Biswas, P.K. (1983). Characteristics of galvanic skin response in anxious patients and normal subjects. *Indian Journal of Clinical Psychology, 10(1),* 159-164.

Chattopadhyay, P.K., Biswas, P.K. & Basu, A.K. (1979). Behaviour therapy in Writers' Cramp : A case report. *Indian Medical Journal, 73(4),* 56-58.

Chattopadhyay, P.K., Bond, A. J. & Lader, M.H. (1975). Characteristics of galvanic skin response in Anxiety States. *Journal Psychiatric Research, 12,* 265-270.

Chattopadhyay, P.K. Cooke, E., Toone, B. & Lader, M. (1980). Habituation of physiological responses in Anxiety. *Biological Psychiatry, 15(5),* 711-723.

Chattopadhyay, P.K. & Chattopadhyay, B. (2008). *Schizophrenia : A look through Indian Culture.* New Age International, New Delhi.

Chattopadhyay, P.K. & Das, M. (1982). Arousal in menstruation : A study with some ANS measures. *Indian Journal of Clinical Psychology, 9(1),* 11-17.

Chattopadhyay, P.K. Dasgupta S. & Laha, H. (1982). Physiological & Psychological aspects of Anxiety in psychiatric patients and normal subjects. *Indian Journal of Psychiatry, 24(2),* 159-163.

Chattopadhyay, P.K., De, S. & Biswas, D. (1993). Impact of parental deprivation on Ego Functioning : An experimental study. *Indian Journal of Clinical Psychology, 20(2),* 63-68.

Chattopadhyay, P.K., Majumder, P. (1982). Physiologic and self-report indices of arousal in Tension Headache sufferers. *Indian Psychologists, 1(1),* 56-60.

Chattopadhyay, P.K., Majumder, P. & Basu, A.K. (1982). Habituation of electrodermal responses in Tension Headache sufferers and Non-Ten on Headache controls. *Indian Journal of Psychiatry, 24(1),* 61-65.

Chattopadhyay, P.K., Mallick, N.B. & Spielberger, C.D. (1984). Adaptation of the State-Trait Anxiety Inventory for Bengali students. In C.D. Spielberger & R. Diazguevrero (Eds.), *Cross Cultural Anxiety,* Vol. II, Chapter 10, Hemisphere Publishing Co., New York.

Chattopadhyay, P.K., Som, B. & Mukhopadhyay, P. (1995). Air pollution and health hazards in human subjects. *Journal of Experimental Psychology, 15,* 327-331; Academic Press, London.

Cheatham, H. (1990). Empowering Black families. In H. Cheatham & J. Stewart (Eds.), *Black families,* New Brunswick, N J : Transaction Press.

Cheek, D. (1976). *Assertive Black... Puzzled White.* San Luis, Obispo, CA : Impact.

Chen, C. (1995). Counselling applications of RET in a Chinese Cultural context. *Journal Rational Emotive & Cognitive Behaviour Therapy, 13,* 117-129.

Cohen, S. & Edwards, J.R. (1989). Personality chracteristics as moderators relationship between stress and disorder. In R.W.J. Newfeld (Ed.), *Advances in the Investigation of Psychological Stress.* New York : Wiley, pp. 235-283.

Conway, N. & Briner, R.B. (2005). *Understanding psychological contracts at work : A critical evaluation of theory and research.* New York : Oxford University Press, Inc.

Crouter, A.C., Bumpus, M.F., Maguire, M.C., & McHale, S.M. (1999). Linking parents' work pressure and adolescents' well-being insights into dynamics in dual-earner families. *Developmental Psychology, 35,* 1453-1461.

Dallman, M.F., Bhatnagar, S. & Vian, V. (2000). Hypothalo-pituitary-adrenal axis. In G. Fink (Ed.), *Encyclopaedia of Stress,* Vol. 2, pp. 468-476, San Diago : Academic Press.

Das, R.C. (1984). The Gita Profile of Ideal Personality. *Psychological Report, 64,* 1074.

Das, M. & Chattopadhyay, P.K. (1982). Arousal in menstruation : A study with some CNS measures. *Indian Journal of Clinical Psychology, 9(2),* 99-104.

Dave, I. (1991). *The basic essentials of counselling.* Sterling Publishers Pvt. Ltd., New Delhi.

Davis, M., Eshelman, E. & McKay, M. (1995a). *The relaxation and stress reduction workbook,* 4th ed., Oakland, CA : New Harbinger.

Davis, M., Robbins, E. & McKay, M. (1995b). *The relaxation and stress management workbook,* 4th ed., Oakland, CA : New Harbinger.

Davis, M.C., Matthews, K.A., Meilahn, E.N. & Kiss, J.E. (1995). Are job characteristics related to fibrinogen levels in middle aged woman? *Health Psychology, 14,* 310-318.

deEsch, J. (1991). Enhanced Therapeutic Skills : Family and ethnic dynamics. Part II, *Paper presented at the North Atlantic Association for Counsellor Education & Supervision,* Albany, NY.

delCamp, R. (2007). Psychological contract violations : An individual difference perspective. *International Journal of Management, 24,* 43-52.

Dhairyam, D. (1961). Research need for development of psychotherapy. In T.K. Menon (Ed.), *Recent trends in psychology.* Orient Longman : New Delhi.

Dhar, R.L. (2009). Cynicism in the Indian IT orgnizations : An exploration of the Employees' perspective. *Qualitative Sociology Review, 5(1),* 152-175.

Dryden, W. (1996). A rose by another name : A personal view on the differences among professional titles. In L. James & S. Palmer (Eds.),*Professional therapeutic titles : Myths and realities. British Psychology Social Division of Counselling Psychology, Occasional Papers, Vol. 2,* Leicester, BPS.

Dutta Ray, S. (1996). *The practice of psychotherapy.* New Age International Publishers Ltd., New Delhi.

Egan. G. (1994). *The skilled helper.* 5th Edn., Pacific Grove, CA : Brooks/Cole.

Einzig, H. (1989). *Counselling & psychotherapy : Is it for me?* British Association for Counselling, Rugby : London.

Ellis, A. (1962). *Reason and emotion in psychotherapy. New York :* Lyle Stuart.

Ellis, A. (1971). *Growth through reason.* Palo Alto, CA : Science & Behaviour Books.

Ellis, A. (1983). The origins of rational-emotive therapy (RET). *Voices, 18,* 29-33.

Ellis, A. (1994). *Reason and emotion in psychotherapy,* New York : Birthlaw.

Ellis, A. (1995). Thinking Process involved in irrational believes and their disturbed consequences. *Journal of Cognitive Psychotherapy, 9,* 105-116.

Flowrian, V., Mikulincer, M. & Taubman, O. (1995). Does hardiness contribute to mental health during a stressful real-life situation : The roles of appraisal of coping. *Journal of Personality and Social Psychology, 68,* 687-695.

Folkman, S. (1997). Positive psychological states and coping with severe stress. *Social Science & Medicine, 45,* 1207-1221.

Frances, A., First, M.B. & Pincus, H.A. (1995). *DSM–IV, Handbook of Differential Diagnosis,* Washington, D.C., American Psychiatric Press.

Frankl, V.E. (1959). *Man's search for meaning.* New York : Pocket Books.

Frankl, V.E. (1985). *The unheard cry for meaning : Psychotherapy and humanism.* New York : Simon & Schuster.

Friedman, H.S., Tucker, J.S., Schwartz, J.E. *et al* (1995). Psychological and behavioural predictors of longevity : the aging and death of the "Termittes". *American Psychologists, 50,* 59-71.

Friedman, M. & Rosenman, R.H. (1974). *Type A behaviours and your heart.* New York : Knopf.

Funk, S.C. (1992). Hardiness : A review of theory and research. *Health Psychology, 11,* 335-345.

Gaur, C.B., Murthy, A. & Nathawat, S.S. (2001). Intelligence and scholastic achievement as determinants of stress & adjustment in adolescent male and female students. *Indian Journal of Clinical Psychology, 28(2),* 257-263.

Gendlin, E. & Hendricks, M. (1978). Changes. In E. Gendlin, *Focussing* (pp.118-144). New York : Everest House.

Gerrig, R.J. & Zimbardo, P.G. (2005). *Psychology and Life.* 7th Edn., Dorling Kindersley (India) Pvt. Ltd., New Delhi.

Ghorpade, M.B. & Kumar, V. (1988). *Introduction to Modern Psychotherapy,* Himalaya Publishing House : Mumbai.

Gillingan, C. (1982). *In a different voice.* Cambridge, MA : Harvard University Press.

Goleman, R. (1971). Meditation as a metatherapy : Hypothesis toward a proposed fifth state of consciousness. *Transpersonal Psychotherapy, 3,* 1-25.

Gray, S.W. & Zide, M.R. (2008). *Psychopathology,* Thompson, Canada, USA.

Gunderson, J.G. (1983). DSM-III Diagnosis of Personality Disorders. In J. Forsch (Ed.), *Cultural perspectives on personality disorders.* Washington, D.C., American Psychiatric Press.

Gustad, J.W. (1953). The definition of counselling. In R.F. Berdie (Ed.), *Role and relationships in counselling,* Minnesota Studies in Student Personnel Work. No. 13, Minneapolis, University of Minnesota Press.

Hale, A.S. & Pinninti, N.R. (1994). Excorcism—Resistant : Ghost Possession treated with Clopenthiazol. *British Journal of Psychiatry, 165,* 396-398.

Harvie-Clark (1999). There are real differences between counselling and psychotherapy. In Feltham, C. (Ed.), *Controversies in Counselling and Psychotherapy,* SAGE : New Delhi.

Hecker, J.E. & Thorpe, G.L. (2005). *Introduction to Clinical Psychology : Science, Practice and Ethics,* Pearson Education, Singapore.

Hoch, E.M. (1963). *Psychotherapy in India : Indo-Asian Culture 12,* Indian Council of Cultural Relations, New Delhi.

Hoch, E.M. (1977). Psychotherapy for Illiterates. In Aritie & Ghrzamonski (Eds.), *New Dimensions in Psychiatry,* Vol. 2, John Wiley, New York.

Holroyd, K.A., Appel, M.A. & Andrasik, F. (1983). A cognitive behavioural approach to psychophysiological disorders. In D. Meichenbaum & M.E. Jaremko (Eds.), *Stress Reduction and Prevention,* New York : Plenum.

Ivey, A.E., Ivey, M.B. & Morgan, L.S. (1997). *Counselling and psychotherapy : A multicultural perspective.* Allyn & Bacon, London.

Jacobs, M. (1988). *Psychodynamic Counselling in Action,* SAGE, London.

Jacobs, M. (1996). Suitable clients for counselling and psychotherapy. *Self and Society, 24(5),* 3-7.

Jacobson, E. (1938). *Progressive relaxation,* 2nd edn., Chicago University, Chicago Press.

Kabat-Zinn, J. (1990). *Full catastrophe living,* New York : Delta.

Kakar, S. (1981). *The inner world* (2nd edn.), Delhi, Oxford University Press, New Delhi.

Kala, A.K. & Wig, N.N. (1982). Delusions across cultures, *Journal of Social Psychiatry, 28,* 185-193.

Kantrowitz, R. & Ballon, M. (1992). A feminist critique of cognitive-behavioural therapy. In L. Brown & M. Ballon (Eds.), *Theories of Personality and Psychopathology : Feminist reappraisals.* New York : Guilford.

Kaplan, J.H., Sadock, B.J. & Grebb, J.A. (1994). *Synopsis of psychiatry,* Baltimore, Williams & Wilkins.

Kapur, M., Barnabas, I., Reddy, M.V. *et al* (1994). Development of a check-list for assessment of childhood pathology in the Indian settings. *Indian Journal of Clinical Psychology, 21,* 40-52.

Kapur, R., Rao, M. & Dalal, M. (1994). A comparative study of prevalence and pattern of psychological disturbances of adolescent boys and girls. *Journal of Personality and Clinical Studies, 10*, 65-70.

Kar, W., Pandey, M., Misra, P., Sengupta, J. & Das, I. (1996). Risk factors of adolescent suicide attempt. *Journal of Eastern Zone of Branch of Indian Psychiatric Society, I(vi)*, 17-22.

Kobasa, S.C. (1970). Stressful life events and health : An inquiry into hardiness. *Journal of Personality and Social Psychology*, 37, 1-11.

Kobasa, S.C. & Puccetti, M.C. (1983). Personality and social resources in stress resistance. *Journal of Personality and Social Psychology, 45*, 839-850.

Kolb, L.C. (1973). *Modern Clinical Psychiatry*, Saunders, London.

Kumaraiah, V. (1980). EMG biofeedback and progressive muscular relaxation in treatments of tension headache. *Indian Journal of Clinical Psychology, 7*, 1-4.

Lader, M.H. & Wing, L. (1981). *Physiological measures, sedative drugs and morbid anxiety*. Oxford University Press, London, Toronto.

Lazarus, A. (1981). *The practice of multi-modal psychotherapy*, New York : McGraw-Hill.

Lazarus, R.S. (1968). Emotions and adaptation : Conceptual and empirical relations. In W. Arnold (Ed.), Nebraska Symposium on Motivation (pp. 175-266), Lincoln University of Nebraska Press.

Lazarus, R.S. & Folkman, S. (1984). *Stress, appraisal, and coping*. New York : Springer.

Lee, C. (1996). Implications for indigenous healing systems. In D. Sue, A. Ivey & Pederson (Eds.), *Toward a theory of multicultural counselling and therapy.* Pacific Grove, CA : Brooks/Cole.

Learner, H. (1992). The limits of phenomenology : A feminist critique of the humanistic personality theories. In L. Brown & M. Ballon (Eds.), *Theories of personality and psychopathology*, New York : Guilford.

Leiter, M.P. & Maslach, C. (2001). Burnout and health. In A. Baum, T.A. Revenson, & J.E. Singer (Eds.), *Handbook of Health Psychology*, pp. 415-426, Mahwah, NJ : Erlbaum.

Leka, S. & Griffith, A. (2005). *Work, Organization & Stress.* Systematic Problem Approaches for Employers, Managers and Trade Union Representatives, Protecting Workers' Health Series No. 3, Institute of Work, Health & Organizations, University of Nottingham, U.K.

Lepine, J.A., Erez, A. & Johnson, D.E. (2002). The nature and dimensionality of organizational citizenship behaviour : a critical review and meta-analysis. *Journal of Applied Psychology, 87*, 52-65.

Lepore, S.J., (1995). Cynicism, social support and cardiovascular reactivity. *Health Psychology, 14*, 210-216.

Lester, S.W., Turnely, W.H., Bloodgood, J.H. & Bolino, M.C. (2002). Not seeing eye to eye : Differences in supervisor and subordinate perceptions of and attributions for psychological contract breach. *Journal of Organizational Behaviour, 23*, 39-56.

Levinson, H. (1965). Reciprocation : The relationship between man and organization. *Administrative Science Quarterly, 9*, 370-390.

Lundberg, U. (2000). Catecholamines. In G. Fink (Ed.), *Encyclopaedia of Stress*, pp. 408-413, San Diego, Academic Press.

Lewis, E.C. (1970). *The psychology of counselling*, New York : Holt, Rinehart & Winston.

Liberman, M., Yalom, I. & Miles, E. (1972). *Encounter groups : First facts.* New York : Basic Books.

MacDougall, J.M., Dembroski, T.M. & Krantz, D.S. (1981). Effects of types of challenge on pressor and heart rate response in Type A and B women. *Psychophysiology, 18*, 1-9.

Maddi, S.R. & Kobasa, S.C. (1984). *The Hardy Executive*, Hillsdale, IL : Dow Jones-Irwin.

Mahoney, M. & Freeman, A. (1985). *Cognition and psychotherapy*, New York : Plenum.

Malhotra, S., Mahotra, S. & Basu, D. (1999). A comparison of the beliefs of Indian alcohol dependent patients and their close family members in their reasons for relapse. *Addiction, 94*, 709-713.

Mallick, N.B., Ghosh, K.K. & Chattopadhyay, P.K. (1986). Hormonal and psychological changes in adolescent boys. *Journal of Psychological Research, 30(3)*, 165-169.

Marks, I., (1978). Behavioural psychotherapy of Adult neurosis. In S.L. Garfiel & Bergin, A.E. (Eds.), *Handbook of Psychotherapy & Behavioural Changes*, John Wiley : New York.

Maslach, C., Schaufell, W.B. & Leiter, M.P. (2001). Job Burnout. *Annual Review of Psychology, 52*, 397-422.

Mason, J.W. (1974). Specificity in the organisation of neuroendocrine response profiles. In P. Seeman & G.M. Brown (Eds.), Frontiers in neurology and neuroscience research. *First International Symposium of the Neuroscience Institute.* Toronto : Canada, University of Toronto.

Mason, J.W. (1975). A historical review of the stress field. *Journal of Human Stress, 1*, 22-36.

Masroorjahan. Haque-Nizamie, S. & Khalique, A. (2002). Efficiency of Luria-Nebraska Neuropsychological Battery in identifying cognitive deficit in epileptic patients. *Indian Journal of Clinical Psychology, 29(2)*, 130-135.

Matthews, K.A. (1982). Psychological perspectives on the Type A behaviour pattern. *Psychological Bulletin, 91*, 293-323.

May, R. (1969). *Love and Will*, New York : Random House.

Meher, B. (1970). *Introduction to Research in Psychopathology*, McGraw-Hill, New York.

Meichenbaum, D. (1991). Evolution of cognitive behaviour therapy. In J. Zeig (Ed.), *The evolution of psychology II*, New York : Brunner/Mazel.

Meichenbaum, D. (1994). *A clinical handbook/practical therapy manual for assessing and treating adults with post-traumatic stress-disorder* (PTSD). Waterloo, Ontario : Institute Press.

Meichenbaum, D.H. & Turk, D. (1982). Stress, coping and disease. A Cognitive-behavioural perspective. In R.W.J. Neufield (Ed.), *Psychological Stress and Psychopathology*, pp. 289-306, New York, McGraw-Hill.

Meninger, K. (1958). *Theory of Psychoanalytic Techniques*, New York : Basic Books.

Michael, A., Mirza, K.A.H., Mukundan. C.R. & Channabasavanna, S.M. (1993). Interhemispheric electroencephalographic coherence as a biological marker in alcoholism. *Acta. Psychiatrica, Scandanavika, 87*, 213-217.

Miller, W.R. & Martin, E.J. (1988). *Behavioural Approaches to Change*, SAGE : London.

Millon, T. (1969). *Modern Psychopathology : A biological approach to maladaptive learning and practicing*. Saunders, New York.

Mishra, B.P., Nizamie, A.H., Shukla, T.R. *et al.* (2000). Luria-Nebraska Neuropsychological Battery—A construct validation study in India. *Indian Journal of Clinical Psychology, 27(2)*, 273-299.

Mishra, G. (1984). *Towards a cognitive model of human motivation. UGC Seminar on Recent Developments in Experimental Psychology.* Dayal Bag Institute of Education, Agra.

Mishra, G. (1988). Relevance of Indian thought to contemporary psychology. In F.M. Sahoo (Ed.), *Psychology in Indian Context*, National Psychological Corporation, Agra.

Mishra, G. & Agarwal, R. (1985). The meaning of achievements, implications for a cross-cultural theory of achievement. In A.R. Langaness & Y.H. Porting (Eds.), *From a different perspective : Studies of behaviour across culture.* Lisse, Swetes & Zetlinger.

Mishra, G., Sahoo, F.M. & Puhan, B.N. (1999). Cultural bias in testing in India. *Review of Applied Psychology, 47(41)*, 309-316.

Mitra, T., Bandyopadhyay, G.K. & Chattopadhyay, P.K. (2002). Variability issues in anxiety ratings in a double-blind study. *Indian Journal of Clinical Psychology, 29(2)*, 136-143.

Mohanty, A., Das, B.S., Mukundan, C.R. & Jamuna, N. (1993a). Cognitive outcome of quality of life after aneurismal subarchnoid haemorrage, Part I. *NIMHANS Journal, 11*, 107-111.

Mohanty, A., Das, B.S., Mukundan, C.R. & Jamuna, N. (1993b). Cognitive outcome of quality of life after aneurismal subarchnoid haemorrage, Part II. *NIMHANS Journal, 11*, 119-124.

Moos, R.H. (1984). Context and coping : Toward a unifying conceptual framework. *American Journal of Community Psychology, 12*, 5-25.

Mukhopadhyay, P., Basu, S. & Chattopadhyay, P.K. (1994). Biofeedback as a therapeutic intervention technique in the treatment of mental disorders. *Indian Journal of Physiology & Allied Sciences, 48(I), 14-20.*

Mukhopadhyay, P. & Chattopadhyay, P.K. (1994). Physiological and endocrinological characteristics of Idiopathic Infertility. *Indian Journal of Clinical Psychology, 21(2)*, 12-19.

Mukhopadhyay, P., & Chattopadhyay, P.K. (1995). LIV in psychophysiological research : The concept revisited. *Social Science International, 11(1 & 2)*, 1-9.

Mukhopadhyay, P., & Chattopadhyay, P.K. (1997). Stress hormone and electrodermal response habituation as diagnostic indices in Idiopathic Infertility. *Indian Journal of Clinical Psychology, 24(2)*, 117-121.

Mukhopadhyay, P., & Chattopadhyay, P.K. (2000). Menstrual distress and self-regulation : An exprimental approach. *Indian Journal of Clinical Psychology, 27(1)*, 104-111.

Mukhopadhyay, P., De, S., Chattopadhyay, P.K. & Biswas, D. (1996). Deprivation : Its impact on arousal modulation and adjustment : A psychophysiological approach. *Indian Journal of Clinical Psychology, 23(2), 161-169.*

Mukhopadhyay, P., & Turner, R.M. (1997). Biofeedback treatment of essential hypertension. *Social Science International, 13*, 1-9.

Munck A. (2000). Corticosteroid and stress. In G. Fink (Ed.), *Encyclopaedia of Stress.* Vol. 1, pp. 570-577, San Diego, Academic Press.

Nathawat, S.S., & Khan, S. (1995). A study of subjective well being of OSHO's devotees. *Indian Journal of Clinical Psychology, 11(1)*, 5-9.

Nayak, A.K. (1997). *Guidance and Counselling*, APH Publishing Corpn., New Delhi.

Naylor-Smith, A. (1994). Counselling and psychotherapy : Is there a difference? *Counselling 5(4)*, 284-286.

Neki, J.S. (1973a). Psychotherapy in India : Past, Present & Future. *American Journal of Psychotherapy, 29*, 92-100.

Neki, J.S. (1973b). Guru-Chela relationship. The possibility of a therapeutic paradigm. *American Journal of Orthopsychiatry, 3*, 755-756.

Neki, J.S. (1976). Cultural relativism of dependence as a dynamic of social and therapeutic relationship. *British Journal of Medical Psychology.*

Neki, J.S. (1977). Dependence : Cross cultural consideration of dynamics. In : A. Arioti & G. Chrzanowski (Eds.), *New dimensions in psychiatry*, John Wiley, New York.

Neki, J.S. (1979), *Psychotherapy in India : Traditions and trends in psychotherapeutic process.* In Kapur, M., Murthy, H.N., Satyavathi, K. & Kapur, R.L. (Eds.), NIMHANS, Bangalore.

Nietzel, M.T., Speltz, M.L., McCauley, E.A. & Bernstein, D.A. (1998). *Abnormal Psychology*, Boston : Allyn & Bacon.

Nikolaou, I., Tomprou, M. & Vokala, M. (2007). Individual's inducements and the role of personality : Implications for psychological contracts. *Journal of Managerial Psychology, 22*, 649-663.

Nowack, K.M. (1989). Coping style, cognitive hardiness and health status. *Journal of Behavioural Medicine, 12*, 145-158.

Nowack, K.M. & Wimer, S. (2011). *Organizational Stress Management : Survival Strategies for Turbulent Times*, Envisia Learning, pp. 1-12.

O'Brian, M. (1996). Counselling Psychology : Identity vs Identity Diffusion. In I. James & S. Palmar (Eds.), *Professional therapeutic titles : Myths and realities.* British Psychological Society Division Counselling Psychology. Occasional Papers, Vol. 2, Leicester, BPS.

O'Hanlon, W. & Weiner-Davis (1989). In Search of Solutions. New York : Norton.

Okun, B. (1992). Object relation and self-psychology : Overview and feminist perspective. In L. Brown & M. Ballou (Eds.), *Theories of Personality and Psychopathology : Feminist reappraisals.* New York : Guilford.

Ollendick, T.H. & King, N.K. (1994). Diagnosis, assessment and treatment of internalizing problems in children : The role of longitudinal data. *Journal Consulting & Clinical Psychology, 62*, 918-927.

Paintal, H.K. & Pandey, N. (1996). A conflict-based study of attitudes of adolescents towards their parents : Implications for parental counselling. *Indian Journal of Clinical Psychology, 23(1)*, 4-11.

Palmer, S. (2000). *Introduction to Counselling and Psychotherapy : The Essential Guide*, SAGE : London.

Pande, S.K. (1968). The Mystique of Western Psychotherapy : An Eastern Interpretation. *Journal of Nervous & Mental Disorders, 146*, 422-432.

Paranjee, A.C. (1984). *Theoretical Psychology : The mention of East and West*, Plenum Press, New York.

Patel, V. (2000). The need for treatment evidence for common mental disorders in developing countries. *Psychological Medicine, 28*, 135-143.

Patterson, C.H. (1973). *Theories of Counselling and Psychotherapy*, New York : Harper & Row.

Pavlov, I.P. (1927). *Conditioned reflex : An investigation of the physiological activity of the cerebral cortex*, London.

Perls, F. (1969). *Gestalt Therapy Verbatim.* Moab, UT : Real People Press.

Perry, Jenkins. M., Repetti, R.L. & Crouter, A.C. (2001). Work and family in the 1990s. In R.M. Milardo (Ed.), *Understanding families into the new millennium : A decade in review*, pp. 200-217. Minneapolis, M.N. National Council of Family Relations.

Piaget, J. (1985). *The equilibrium of cognitive structure.* Chicago : University of Chicago Press.

Pickering, T.G., Devereux, R.B., James, G.D. *et al* (1996). Environmental influences on blood pressure and the role of job strain. *Journal of Hypertension, 14* (Suppl.), 179-185.

Prasad, R. (1982). *Patanjali Yoga Sutra*, Oriental Books, New Delhi.

Prasad, M. (1997). Registration of Clinical Psychologists. *Indian Journal of Clinical Psychology, 24(1)*, 3-6.

Puhan, B.N. (1982). *Issues in Psychological Assessment*, National Psychological Corporation, Agra, India.

Puhan, B.N. (1995). Projective inventory : An indigenous approach to personality assessment. *Psychological & Developmental Societies*, 7, 115-131.

Raghuram, A., Venkateswaran, A., Ramkrishnan, J. & Weiss. M.G. (2002). Traditional community resource for mental health : A report of temple healing from India. *British Medical Journal, 325*, 38-40.

Raja, U., Johns, G. & Nitalian, S.N. (2004). The impact of personality on psychological contracts. *Academy of Management Journal, 47(3)*, 350-367.

Ramdas (Baba) (1971). *Be here now.* New York : Crown.

Rangaswami, K. (1991). Child rearing practices in changing context in India. *Indian Journal of Psychological Medicine, 14(1)*, 95-96.

Rangaswami, K. (1994), Spirituality and psychotherapy (Editorial). *Indian Journal of Clinical Psychology, 21*, 1.

Rangaswami, K. (1996). Indian system of psychotherapy. *Indian Journal of Clinical Psychology, 23(1)*, 62-75.

Rao, S.N. (1964), Problems of adjustment and academic achievement. *Journal of Vocational & Educational Guidance, 10*, 66-79.

Rao, S.N. (1965a). Causes of student failure. *Symposium on Student Failure. Indian Science Congress Association.*

Rao, S.N. (1965b). *Student personnel services in India.* University of Minnesota & Associated Research Councils, Washington, D.C.

Rao, S.N. (1966). Culture and mental disorders : A study in an Indian Mental Hospital. *Indian Journal of Social Psychiatry, 12*, 2-3.

Rao, S.N. (1967a). Adjustment problems of college students. *Journal of Vocational & Educational Guidance, 13*, 83-92.

Rao, S.N. (1967b). *Student performance and adjustment.* S.V. University, Tirupati, India.

Rao, S.N. (1969). Psychological factors and student unrest. *Seminar on Student Unrest, Proceedings.* Benaras Hindu University, India.

Rao, S.N. (1970). Scholastic performance and its relation to anxiety. *Proceedings of Indian Academy of Applied Psychology.*

Rao, S.N. (1971). A prognostic study of academic achievement : *Indian Educational Review*, N.C.E.R.T., *6*, 196-213. New Delhi.

Rao, S.N. (1972). A follow-up study of academic achievers and under-achievers in an Engineering College. *Proceedings of Indian Science Congress Association.*

Rao, S.N. (1973). A follow-up study of academic over- and under-achievers. *S.V. University Journal, 2*, 97-103.

Rao, S.N. (1974). Academic anxiety and achievement. *Psychological Studies, 19*, 38-42.

Rao, S.N. (1981). *Counselling Psychology.* Tata McGraw-Hill Publishing Co., New Delhi.

Rao, V.N. & Parthasarathi, R. (1993). Psychological intervention in school settings. *The Andhra Pradesh Journal of Psychological Medicine, 6*, 18-21.

Rau, H., Bührer, M., Wietkunat, R. (2003). Biofeedback of R-wave-to-pulse interval normalizes blood pressure. *Applied Psychophysiology and Biofeedback. 28*, 37-46.

Razaram, G. (1961). The observable unconscious and the inferable conscious in current soviet Psychophysiology : Interoceptive conditioning, semantic conditioning, and the orienting reflex. *Psychological Review, 68*, 81-147.

Reber, A.S. (1985). *Dictionary of psychology.* Penguin Books Ltd., Harmondsworth, Middlesex, England.

Restubog, S.L.D., Bordia, P. & Tang, R.L. (2006). Effects of psychological contract breach on performance of IT employees : The mediating role of affective commitment. *Journal of Occupational and Organizational Psychology, 79*, 299-306.

Reynolds, J.R. (1997). The effects of industrial employment conditions in job-related distress. *Journal of Health and Social Behaviour, 38*, 105-116.

Rigazio-Digilio, S.A., Ivey, A.E., Ivey, M.B. & Simek-Morgan, L. (1997). Developmental counselling and therapy : Individual and family therapy. In Ivey, A., Ivey, M.B. & Simek-Morgan, L. (Eds.). *Counselling & Psychotherapy : A Multicultural Perspective*, 4th Edn., Allyn & Bacon, London.

Robinson, S.L. & Morrison, E.W. (1995). Organizational citizenship behaviour : A psychological contract perspective. *Journal of Organizational Behaviour, 16*, 239-298.

Robinson, S.L. & Morrison, E.W. (2000). Development of psychological contract, breach and violation : A longitudinal study. *Journal of Organizational Behaviour, 21*, 525-546.

Robinson, S.L. & Rousseau, D.M. (1994). Violating the psychological contract : Not the exception but the norm. *Journal of Organizational Behaviour, 15*, 245-259.

Rogers, C. (1942). *Counselling and Psychotherapy.* Mifflin, Houghton, Boston.

Rogers, C. (1957). The necessary and sufficient conditions of therapeutic personality change. *Journal of Consulting Psychology, 21*, 95-103.

Rogers, C. (1961). *On becoming a person.* Mifflin, Boston, Houghton.

Rogers, C. (1962). The interpersonal relationship : The core of guidance. *Harvard Educational Review, 32*, 416-429.

Rousseau, D.M. (2004). Psychological contracts in the workplace : Understanding the ties that motivate. *Academy of Management Executive, 10(1)*, 120-122.

Runk, Bette (2011). What is Biofeedback? National Institute of Mental Health, Division of Scientific and Public Information—Plain Talk Series, Ruth Kay (Ed.), http://www.psychotherapy.com.

Rushing, B., Ritter, C. & Burton, R.P.D. (1992). Race differences in the effects of multiple roles on health : longitudinal evidence from a national sample of older men. *Journal of Health & Social Behaviour, 33*, 126-139.

Sandler, J., Holder, A. & Dave, C. (1970). Basic psychoanalytic concepts : IV. Counter Transference. *British Journal of Psychiatry, 117*, 83-88.

Sanyal, N. (2004). Emotional profile in the context of depression, anxiety, aggression, and adjustment in epileptic and non-epileptic adolescents : A comparative study. *SIS Journal of Projective Psychology & Mental Health, 11*, 105-114.

Sanyal, S., Chattopadhyay, P.K. & Biswas, D. (1998). Electrodermal arousal and self-report indices in patients with somatization disorder. *Indian Journal of Clinical Psychology, 25(2)*, 144-148.

Sarafino, E.P. (1994). *Health psychology : Biopsychological interaction, 2nd ed.*, John Wiley & Sons, Inc., New York.

Sartre, J. (1986). *Being and Nothingness.* London : Metheun.

Scafuza, M. & Kuipers, E. (1999). Coping strategies in relations to people with schizophrenia before and after psychiatric admission. *British Journal of Psychiatry, 174*, 154-158.

Scheier, M.F., Carver, C.S. & Bridges, M.W. (1994). Distinguishing optimism from neuroticism and trait anxiety, self-mastery, and self-esteem. A revaluation of Life Orientation Test. *Journal of Personality and Social Psychology, 67*, 1063-1078.

Schulz, R., Bookwala, J., Knopp, J.E. *et al.* (1996). Pessimism, age and cancer mortality. *Psychology and Aging, 11*, 304-309.

Scorzelli, J. & Reinkee-Scorgelli, M. (1994). Cultural sensitivity and cognitive therapy in India. *Counselling Psychologists, 22*, 603-610.

Scully, J.H. (1996). *Psychiatry.* Baltimore : Williams and Wilkins.

Seeman, T.E., Berkman, L.F., Gulanski, B.L. (1995). Self-esteem and neuroendocrine response to challenge : MacAurther Studies of Successful Aging. *Journal of Psychosomatic Research, 39*, 69-84.

Selye, M. (1956). *The Stress of Life*, New York : McGraw-Hill.

Selye, M. (1976). *Stress in Health & Disease*, Philadelphia, Lippincott.

Sethi, B.B. (1977). Need for an Indian psychotherapeutic model (Editorial), *Indian Journal of Psychology, 19(1)*, 1.

Siegel, J.M. (1993). Companion animals : In sickness and in health. *Journal of Social Issues, 49*, 157-167.

Shamasundar, G. (1979). What kind of psychotherapy in the Indian setting? *Indian Journal of Psychiatry, 21*, 31-33.

Shenoy, J. & Kapur, M. (1995). Sensitivity of the behaviour problem scale of the child behaviour check-list in an Indian Clinical sample. *Indian Journal of Clinical Psychology, 22(2)*, 43-49.

Sinha, D. (1981). Non-Western perspectives in Psychology : Why, What and Whether. *Indian Journal of Clinical Psychology, 3*, 1-9.

Sinha, D. (1983). Human assessment in the Indian context. In S.H. Irvine & J.W. Berny (Eds.), *Human assessments and cultural facto.* Pelinum Press, New York.

Sinha, D. (1984). Reactions on measurement of human motivation in India. *Psychological Studies, 29(3)*, 199-206.

Sinha, D. (1986). *Psychology in the Third World Country—The Indian Experience.* SAGE Publications, New Delhi.

Sinha, D. & Holtzman, W.H. (1984). The impact of psychology on the Third World Development. *Indian Journal of Psychology* (Special Issues), *19(2)*, 15-20.

Sinha, U.K. & Kapur, M. (2001). Pattern and prevalence of emotional disturbances in Indian adolescent boys. *Indian Journal of Clinical Psychology, 28(2)*, 209-215.

Sinha, V.K. (2000). Academic stress and its management. In S. Gupta (Eds.), *Proceedings of the Orientation Course in Clinical Psychology,* IIMS, New Delhi.

Smith, E.E., Hoeksema, S., Fredrickson, B. & Loftus, G.R. (2003). *Atkinson and Hilgard's Introduction to Psychology,* 14th edn., Thompson & Wordsworth, U.K., U.S.A.

Smith, T.W. (1992). Hostility and health : Current status of a psychosomatic hypothesis. *Health Psychology, 11*, 139-150.

Snaith, P. (1998). Meditation and Psychotherapy. *British Journal of Psychiatry, 173*, 193-195.

Speca, M., Carlson, L.E., Gooday, E. & Angen, M. (2000). A randomized wait-list controlled clinical trial : The effect of mindfulness meditation based stress reduction programme on mood and symptoms of stress in cancer patients. *Psychosomatic Medicine, 62*, 613-622.

Sridhar, K.R. (1981). *Yoga Therapy in Tension Headache.* Unpublished M.D. Thesis, NIMHANS, Bangalore University.

Srivastava, A.K. & Misra, G. (1996). Changing Perspective in understanding intelligence : An appraisal. *Indian Journal of Abstracts & Reviews, 3*, 3-4.

Srivastava, A.K., Tripathi, A.M. & Misra, G. (1996). The status of intelligence testing in India : A preliminary analysis. *Indian Educational Review, 31(1)*, 1-10.

Strawbridge, S. (1999). Counselling and psychotherapy as enabling and empowering. In C. Feltham (Ed.), *Controversies in Counselling & Psychotherapy,* SAGE, New Delhi.

Sue, D. (1990). Culture-specific strategies in counselling : A conceptual framework. *Professional Psychology, 21*, 424-433.

Suhail, K. (2000). A comparative study of delusions and hallucinations in Indian and White psychiatric patients. *Indian Journal of Clinical Psychology, 27(2)*, 202-208.

Surya, N.C. & Jayaram, S.S. (1964). Some basic considerations of psychotherapy in Indian Setting, *Indian Journal of Psychology, 6*, 153-156.

Sutherland, S.M. & Frances, A. (1995). Avoidant Personality Disorder. In G.O. Gobbard (Ed.). *Treatment of Psychiatric Disorders.* Washington, DC; American Psychiatric Press.

Tamase, K. (1991). The effects of introspective-developmental counselling. *Paper presented at the American Association of Counselling and Development*. Reno. Navada.

Tamase, K. & Kato, M. (1990). *Effect of questions about factual and affective aspects of life events in an introspective interview.* Bull. Nara. University of Education, pp. 153-163.

Taylor, S.E. (1999). *Health Psychology,* pp. 316-317, 4th Edn., Boston, McGraw-Hill, Singapore.

Tekleab, A.G. & Taylor, M.S. (2003). Aren't there two parties in an employment relationship? Antecedents and consequences of organisation—Employee agreement on contract obligations and violations. *Journal of Organizational Behaviour, 24,* 585-608.

Thorne, B.J. (1992a). Psychotherapy and counselling are indistinguishable. In Feltham, C. (Ed.), *Controversies in Psychotherapy and Counselling,* SAGE, New Delhi.

Thorne, B.J. (1992b). Psychotherapy and Counselling : the quest for differences. *Counselling, 3(4),* 242-248.

Thorpe, G.L. & Olson, S.L. (1997). Behaviour therapy : concepts, procedures and application (2nd edn.), Boston : Allyn & Bacon.

Tillich, P. (1971). Existentialism and Psychotherapy. Review of Existential Psychology and Psychiatry, 1, 8-16.

Tomaka, J., Blascovich, J., Kelsey, R.M. *et al* (1993). Subjective, physiological and behavioural effect of threat and challenge appraisal. *Journal of Personality and Social Psychology, 65,* 248-260.

Tseng, W. & McDermott, J. (1981). Culture, mind, and therapy : An introduction to cultural psychiatry. New York, Brunner/Mezel.

Tucker, I.F. (1970). *Adjustment : Models & Mechanisms.* Academic Press, New York.

Tyler, L. (1961). *The work of the counsellor* (2nd Edn.), East Norwalk, CT : Appleton & Lange.

Uchino, B.N. & Garvey, T.S. (1997). The availability of social support reduces cardiovascular reactivity to acute psychological stress. *Journal of Behavioural Medicine, 20,* 15-28.

Udupa, K.N. (1985). *Stress and its management by yoga.* Motilal Banarasidas, Chennai.

Vahia, N.S., Doongaji, D.R., Jeste, D.V., Ravinderanath, S. & Kapoór, M. (1973). Experience with the therapy based on concepts of Patanjali in the treatment of psychiatric disorders. *Indian Journal of Psychiatry, 15,* 32-34.

Vasudevan, A.R., Kumaraiah, V., Mishra, H. & Balodhi, J.P. (1994), Yogic meditation in tension headache. *NIMHANS Journal,* 66-73.

Verma, V.K. (1995). Psychotherapy, Yoga & Meditation, In : S.H. Skoslow, R. Srinivasmurthy & G.V. Coelho (Eds.), *Decade of Brain.* National Institute of Mental Health, Rockville, USA.

Venkatesan, S. (2002a). Extension and validation of Gessels Drawing Test of Intelligence in a group of children with communicating handicaps. *Indian Journal of Clinical Psychology, 29(2),* 173-177.

Venkatesan, S. (2002b). Reappraisal of Bombay-Karnataka version of the Binet-Simon Intelligence Scale (1964). *Indian Journal of Clinical Psychology, 29(1)*, 72-78.

Weinder, G. Boughal, T., Connor, S.L. *et al* (1997). Relationship of job strain to standard coronary risk factors and psychological characteristics in women and men : A family study. *Health Psychology, 16*, 239-247.

Weiten, W. & Lloyd, M.A. (2004). *Psychology applied to modern life.* Thompson Asia Private Limited, Singapore.

Whisman, M.A. & Kwon, P. (1993). Life stress and dysphoria : The role of self-esteem and hopelessness. *Journal of Personality and Social Psychology, 65*, 1054-1060.

White, J. & Praham, T. (1991). *The psychology of Blacks : An African-American perspective*, (2nd Edn.), Englewood Cliffs, NJ : Prentice-Hall.

Williams, P.G., Wiebe, D.J. & Smith, T.W. (1992). Coping processes as mediators of the relationship between hardiness and health. *Journal of Behavioural Medicine, 15*, 237-256.

Williamson, E.G. (1950). *Counselling Adolescents*, New York : McGraw-Hill.

Williamson, E.G. (1965). *Vocational Counselling*, New York : McGraw-Hill.

Winnicott, D. (1988). *Human Nature*, New York : Schockan.

Wolberg, I.R. (1977). *Techniques of psychotherapy.* New York : Grune & Straton. New York.

World Health Organization (1996). *Constitution of the World Health Organization*, Geneva, Switzerland, WHO Basic Documents.

Wyatt, F. (1988). What is clinical psychology? In A.Z. Guiora & M.A. Brandwin (Eds.), *Perspective in Clinical Psychology*, Princeton, NJ, D. Van-Nostrand.

Yamamoto, K. (1963). Counselling psychologists—Who are they? *Journal of Counselling Psychology, 10*, 211-221.

Zarate, R. & Agras, W.S. (1994). Psychosocial treatment of phobia and panic disorders. *Psychiatry, 57(2)*, 133-141.

SUBJECT INDEX

D

R

W

Y

AUTHOR INDEX

Some exciting gifts are up for grabs with this book!!

STRESS IN CORPORATE SECTORS AND CLINICS INDIAN SCENARIO

FREE Gifts Rs. 1000/-

Prabal Kumar Chattopadhyay

Dear Readers

By now you must have gone through this book in the entirety. So we invite your assessment on this title with absolute impartiality and candid observations. After all, we publishers blindly depend on your benchmarking. Friends, please fill up the open spaces below with CAPITAL LETTERS. You may add some extra sheets of paper if the space provided is not sufficient for you.

i. What are the important topics of your syllabus which are not adequately covered in this book?

ii. In which chapters and on what topics the treatment of the subject-matter by the author is not satisfactory and why?

iii. Have you come across the typos, factual inaccuracies, inconsistencies, and other forms of mistakes in the book? If yes, then please specify the mistakes and page numbers.

iv. Name top three books on the same subject, which, in your consideration, are better than this book. Could you provide some reasons?

Your 1st Preference: ....

Your 2nd Preference: ....

Your 3rd Preference: ....

v. Any suggestion to improve the quality of illustrations, diagrams etc.?

vi. How did you like the cover design? Any suggestions on colours?

vii. Suggestions for further improvement of production standard:

viii. Who recommended you this book:

☐ Teacher ☐ Friend ☐ Parents ☐ Bookseller ☐ Librarian

ix. Name of the person who has recommended:

Designation: ....

Address: ....

Phone No.: ....

e-mail: ....

x. Name and address of the bookseller from whom you have purchased this book:

....

....

....

xi. Name and address of the library where you would like to find the book:

....

....

xii. Name and address of your institution (Please mention the University or Board):

....

....

xiii. Your name, e-mail, and complete postal address:

....

....

....

xiv. A few other titles published by us that you would like to read:

....

....

The best assessment will be rewarded half-yearly. The award will be in the form of our publications, as decided by the Editorial and Marketing Operations Division, amounting to Rs. 1000/- (Rupees one thousand) only.

....

Please mail the filled up coupon at your earliest to :

Editorial & Marketing Operations Division

NEW CENTRAL BOOK AGENCY (P) LTD

8/1 Chintamoni Das Lane, Kolkata 700 009

West Bengal, INDIA

Ph. No.: 033 + 22418411, 22418573, 22419094

Fax: 033 + 22419573, 22413852

e-mail: ncbapvtltd@eth.net, ncba@cal2.vsnl.net.in

Website: www.centralgroup.com